This is a gathering of autumn flowers, what has remained of the summer garden, the gathering before the scattering. Poems in the elder's voice, that ripened voice which grows only out of a considered life, from a man who has spent the currency of his seventy some years in deepening that life through the practice of poetry. *Lake Winds* brings us the poetry of appreciation and gratitude. No busy ego racket here. These poems come from a quieter level of mind that trusts that all of this is held within the secret direction/of everything. They acknowledge that truth, in poet Rumi's words, that "Someone has filled the cup before us. It is understood that we must prepare it for those who follow." Each of these poems is a filled cup awaiting a reader.

Consider the lessons of "The Weed by the Garage." Here, the poet hesitates to pull a weed from the garden. "Is it a weed or not/and how are we to decide?" The subtle teachings of Zen whisper here as they do so often throughout. If one is to act compassionately: don't tell me show me. We are cautioned to stop choosing between this and that, to include it all, weed and flower, in Big Mind. Then, the poet offers this extraordinary simple line, a sharpened blade to with which to sever every knot of delusion. "Without judgment, all are dear."

The beautifully spun "Walking a Field into Evening" teaches us the wisdom of letting go.

> No more arguments,
>
> Just heart sense, or talk about nothing.
>
> Take long walks in the woods at dawn or dusk,
>
> Breathe in the damp musty air,
>
> Learn to listen before I die.

These poems speak to those who have learned to listen.
 - Maj Ragain

Other Books by Larry Smith

Fiction:
> *The Free Farn: A Novel* (Bottom Dog Press 2011)
> *The Long River Home: A Novel* (Bottom Dog Press, 2009).
> *Faces and Voices: Tales* (Bird Dog Publishing, 2007).
> *Working It Out* (Ridgeway Press, 1998).
> *Beyond Rust* (Bottom Dog Press, 1995).

Memoirs:
> *Milldust and Roses* (Ridgeway Perss 2002).

Poetry:
> *Each Moment All: Poems as Meditations* (March Street
>   Press/ Bottom Dog Press 2012).
> *Tu Fu Comes to America: A Story in Poems* (March Street Press
>   2010).
> *A River Remains* (WordTech Editions 2006).
> *Thoreau's Lost Journal* (Westron Press 2002).
> *Steel Valley: Postcards & Letters* (Pig Iron Press 1992).
> *Across These States* (Bottom Dog Press 1985).
> *Scissors, Paper, Rock* (Cleveland State Univ. Poetry Center
>   1982).
> *Growth* (Northwoods Press 1975).

Biography:
> *Lawrence Ferlinghetti: Poet-At-Large* (Southern Illinois
>   University Press, 1983).
> *Kenneth Patchen: Rebel Poet in America* (A Consortium
>   of Small Presses, 2000; revised edition Bottom Dog
>   Press, 2013).

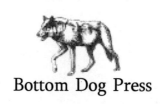

Bottom Dog Press

Lake Winds

Poems

Larry Smith

With love & respect
Larry

Harmony Series
Bottom Dog Press
Huron, Ohio

Bottom Dog Press, Inc.
P.O. Box 425 /Huron, Ohio 44839
http://smithdocs.net

Credits

Cover Photo: Laura Watilo Blake
Interior Photos: Brian Smith & Larry Smith
Author photo by Laura Smith
Cover Design: Susanna Sharp-Schwacke

Acknowledgments

Some of these poems appeared in three chapbooks: *Each Moment All, Waking,* and *Meditations,* and in these magazines: *Yoga Journal International, Pudding Magazine, Everything Stops and Listens, Fellowship,* and *Pine Mountain Sand and Gravel.*

My thanks to the members of the Firelands Writing Center for their continuing support and input, and to my initial readers of this book: Allen Frost, Laura Smith, Susanna Sharp-Schwacke, Maj Ragain, and my good wife Ann Smith for their editing skills and human insights. A special thanks goes to the members of Converging Paths Mediation Center and to friends and family.

Dedication

For Ann
Who lived and loved it with me.

Author's Preface

These poems from the last 10 years are all since the publication of my *A River Remains*. A couple chapbooks came along, but this feels like the big 'last words' collection of an older man. The ancient Chinese poets used the elders's voice, even when much younger. I found or earned it honestly, and am comfortable with the mellow reach of it. Some of these stretch back into memories of youthful times, lost parents and friends and places transformed; many simply open to the nowness of nature, loves, relationships, particularly family including my blessing of children and grandchildren. Most are shared with my loving partner and wife Ann.

My first book of poetry was *Growth*, a coming of age and entering maturity book, followed by one of memoirs in *Milldust and Roses*. The journey of these poems is deeper and more quiet, meditative and contemplative while also staying open to the images and voices around. I have been fortunate to have literature and writing as part of my path, and I've been happy to publish the works of others, whether in books or at community readings. As I say of my years of teaching, "I smile, knowing that/ for all of these years I've been paid/ for doing what I love."

My spiritual path is charted here, which includes an early and humble Christian training, a lifelong bond with Transcendental thought, the non-dualist outlook of Buddhism, and finally my embracing of the heart of Catholic compassion and grace. Sisters Julita and Olivia helped me along this way. I write of my path here, yet with an open mind and heart to the paths of others. As my good friend Bill Wright would say, "May the world be a better place because you lived." Life has truly been a matter of converging paths, and I share mine here.

Summer Evening

I want some old folk song
to wake me into clearness:
banjo singing like rain drops
pounding a tin pan in the yard,
three women on porch steps
turning sounds into the
sweet harmonies of friends,
guitar chording lake wind,
leaves parting again and again.
Our hearts quickening as we
lean into evening light.
May it rain all night long

The River

Sitting on the cabin porch
near my wife and dog,
I hear the gentle surge
of water over rocks—
birds inside the stream.

A quiet day of sun and shade.

Strumming soft guitar chords
to answer the stream's voice,
I melt away.
My path becomes a river
holding all.

(7.3.13 Wagner's cabin)

Nature's Garden

What have you done with the garden
that was entrusted to you?
- Antonio Machado

Tell me,
what is it you plan to do
with your one
wild and precious life?
- Mary Oliver

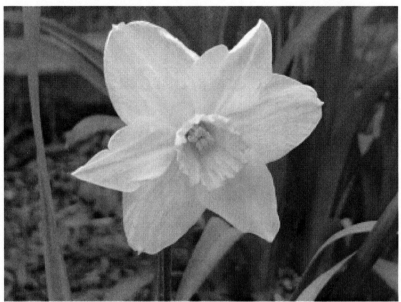

(Photo: Brian Smith)

Morning Blessings

That door knocking may be your own heart.

Morning is always born
out of darkness,
the interior exposed
in silence, giving birth
to life to come—
always a new beginning
original and clean.

Morning call of birds,
branches tapping at windows,
the dog stretches and yawns.
Our eyes open to it
as we bring our dreams
out of darkness and
into light.

Walking into It

Along the lake in morning light,
thought and circumstance come toward me.
This tall wave pushes me back and along,
leaving me stumbling forward, holding air in lungs.
Long I've been walking into it, the sand
unsettling at my feet, pulling me down toward
a stream—a river—this lake of doubt.

Water settles round me again, as gulls
rise from the shore, span out across
a morning sky in wings of flight. And I
stand in windswept lake, bare feet
holding to the earth which I must
trust beneath me.

Beneath a Blue Sky

for Rosa and Maya

At the edge of the lake
smoke blows up river
over the limestone plant.
A great blue heron stands
on a post, then lifts off
into the wind while waves
come splashing over rocks.

It is a day without measure.

No fishermen in mid-October
only a few school children
taking the long way home
turning the cool air to talk.
One walking silent on the shore
presses a rounded stone
into the soft pocket
of her palm.

I and Thou in the Wild

> *No one*
> *walks along this path*
> *this autumn evening.*
>   *-Basho*

The field beside the road
is a block of golden light
amber in the evening sun.
And in the mauve sky
wild geese wing together
        calling each to all
                gliding their way
        homeward.

And so my car glides with them
past mailboxes, driveways, houses
over a country road
where lies a fallen deer,
a heap in the tall grass,
its body tans to reds
all the colors of autumn.

Lake Winds

Ice chunks float down river
pushed out into the land of lake
where South winds shove them
back along the rugged shore.

You cannot walk across
these prehistoric shards
only stare in wonder with
cold air against your face.

Thin shadow of geese
calling overhead.
This wild of Nature held
against the mind's chaos.

Housebound in March

The snow a foot deep
yet March robins and nuthatch
gather at the feeder.

Redwing blackbirds in from fields,
two cardinals among the pines,
scatter at a flock of starlings.

All of this a little film
against a background of white.

I've heard from neighbors that eagles
are browsing the frozen shoreline.

Birdfeeder on Snow Days

I've been looking out at the bird feeder
with its foot of snow and lack of seed.
It's been several days of below zero
with snow mounting up in cones.
So far, I've just been looking out.
The bag of seed bought days ago
still sits by the back door unopened.
Where are the birds anyway? I ask myself.
And will they come if I set out seed?
I trust that they will, but not at first.
Tentative though hungry they will come
to test the trays of snowy seed,
while watching the house for a threat.
But then they will send out word
and the troops will arrive to feed:
ruddy starlings and wizened cardinals,
maybe even a bluejay, or a rare hawk
out to snatch one of these others.
The yard cats have all disappeared,
holed up in basements or garages.
Life is always a risk, and God promises
only acceptance and grace. The rest
is up to us and the fates. Thinking all this,
I rise from the couch to put on my boots.
take the seed out where it's of use.

A Cardinal Arrives

The red bird comes with morning snow
gathering spare seed from yard feeder,
each seed a kernel of hidden heat,
a strength within for the deepening cold.

More quiet flakes come drifting down
covering grass and bushes and feeder.
And where do the birds go? I ask myself and dog
watching through our window glass.
And where do I go when things pile up
and threaten my nesting place?

The cardinal shows no signs of fear
plucking seeds in a steady glide
of back and forth to tree branch
safe inside the weather.

The Starlings

Along the road
a flock of small wild birds
rises in a great cloud…like leaves
blown in wind, turning like
music across the page, and we
pass into or through them—
our eyes open, hearts beating
to be inside this storm of
wildness, this winging body
of wordless beings.

Meditation on Birds and Water

Seagulls gather in herds of hundreds
along the shoreline at dusk,
standing in mute meditation
they look out across the lake
inside the sound of wind and waves.

And when the light fades
to almost dark, sunset
sinking into the waters...
At once they all rise,
hover a moment, then gently
glide eastward above the waters—
the sky more birds than clouds now—
waves of them winging before us
seated in sand and wonder.
To see and know within
this silent significance
beyond words and thought:
waves pounding on the shore
birds flying together at dusk
day moving softly into night.

Breaking the Silence

Awake before the others
in my sister's house,
I step the quiet boards
of the back deck inside
the stillness of the dawn.
At the back edge of yard
a stand of trees rise thick and deep
without movement.

Wild turkey and deer
run here some days,
but not this morning.
Here a gentle silence
covers everything
before day's awakening.

Inside asleep: my wife,
my sister and her husband.
I stand alone in morning
till I hear the dogs
tapping at the glass door.
I slide it open
and three dogs glide past,
then pant at my feet before
heading down into the yard.

Inside the dawn's silence
I drift alone and still,
until a high sharp bird calls:
kwirr—kwirr—kwirr—
a shrill alarm.
My eyes search among the leaves
of the old oak—nothing.
And the call comes again:
kwirr—kwirr—kwirr—
followed now by a quick:
tap—tap—tapping…Awaken!
At last I see him—red capped
and with black barred coat,
the worker up with the sun
and opening our day.

The Rescuing

*"Last night's rain
has soaked the sandy beach.
The spring wind blows
against the currents."* –Tu Fu

Birds chirp to each other
in this morning's trees,
as I sit on the back porch
awaiting my wife.

Yesterday a robin came down
our chimney into the fireplace;
trapped by fate or accident,
we all wanted her free.

My wife and I crouched near the
screen, plotting her release, yet
each time we dared to reach in
she hopped back under the grate.

So hard to help sometimes,
her fears and our urgings
could prove tragic.
Reason only taking us so far
we tried to sense...a trapped bird...

then hung a blanket over the screen
so light was just from above.
An hour later—still there,
her feathers covered now with ash.
We kneeled again, and reaching in
I swept a small broom across
while Ann lurched over with cloth
forcing the moment. She hopped out,
Ann dropped the towel
gently folding her inside,
then lifting her out, while I
rushed to open the door.

Setting her down in the wet grass,
Ann rose, moved back. The robin hopped
looked about stunned to be free at last.
We too watched at our screen door
till out of nowhere another robin came
to nudge our friend to flight, and
Ann with tears breathed out,
"I was so afraid to hurt
so tender a thing."

Along the Edge

Tall grass, winter brown, and the wind
blowing steady along the lake. Gulls
come flying close across the waters. Firm
sand beneath my feet, as my dog and I
look out toward what must be Canada.
The line of sea and sky blue-gray
melts into a blur of white. The dog runs
to lick the waters, steady swish of lake over land.
And as she turns to read my face, I sense
this sweet convergence of detail.
Central or ephemeral depends upon
how we see and hold this moment,
how we stand in this wild labyrinth
beyond geometry and measure.
The dog trots back to nuzzle
her head against my palm.

Abiding the Weather

The lake rolls in with March winds,
dark peaks and white foam tumbling on,
pouring over rocks to shore.

My own breath close in my chest,
my heart restless and longing
perhaps to sleep.

Rain falls against my face,
a wetness of emotion
penetrating my body shelter.

Weather always surprises, no way to
predict or control, wait and see
what comes—then make do.

I've left the dog at the house
sleeping on her cushion.
I take a breath and walk myself home.

Watching Things Move

After Denise Levertov

When I walk the street
I notice old leaves
nestled together along
mute curbs.

My presence does not matter.

Imperceptibly they move along
as street elders, their aged
bodies touching, their
voices longing to rest.

Waking while walking
I sense the way life flows:
sun into moon, waves
inside of waves, water and wind,
each day ever falling
into night.
We sleep
to rise again.

Grace of the Day

My little dog trots along beside me
treading the street toward the lake.

Late afternoon sun casts shadows
we walk through, without a plan
or worry, moving along like the
gulls above in clear blue skies.

When I stop, she does.
When I start, she begins,
trusting the road and me.
And I trusting her to bring
me home again.

Walking Autumn

A white moon at noon still
high above the courthouse clock.
Below a garden of mums
welcomes the sun, so
warm on our backs.
"Fall equinox," my wife says
taking my arm, while I nod.
Our path ever before us
and behind.

A black dog trots across the wet grass
running toward us, his bark
more a greeting than threat.

Pulling Wild Thistle

We work for hours
at my son's house
trimming grass, pulling weeds.
The thistle are taller
than my grandsons
who run about the yard
raking leaves, chasing our dog,
at noon, bringing drinks.

Sharp thorns cut through
my gloves, yet I grip
their green stems down
near the white roots
then tug them out
one by one,
laying them straight
like fallen troops
dying in noonday sun.

Was it kindness or neglect
that allowed this growth?
Am I destroyer or savior
killing what's wild
in the name of order?

The palms of my hands
will sting with my deeds
for hours.

The Weed by the Garage

Near my wife's hydrangeas
and Black-eyed Susans,
a green stalk protrudes.
Its leafy stem in August sun
feathers out against the
house's blue siding.
A stranger among friends
at a garden party.

Its simple beauty brings on
my quiet laugh.
Is it a weed or not
and how do we decide?
"Don't tell me, show me,"
the Buddhist priest commands.

I bend to stroke it.

Without judgment, all are dear.
This green straggler serves
as food and home to insects,
and in this moment
awakens me.

The Visit

Six days spent out West
at our daughter's house
near rocky forests
along Bellingham Bay.

I soon find my way
to the Co-op coffeeshop,
rich smell of foods, broad
windows looking out at rain.

I've brought a book
and so begin to read,
spreading my mind
over currents of words.

Today she tells us
we will drive up Mt. Baker,
take an off-road trail
into the forest. And so

we travel wooded roads,
abandon their Volvo and
hike along a rushing stream
spilling over rounded boulders—
sharp scent of pines and cedar.

Her dog leaps the logs
which we walk around.
Her children toss rocks
into the bounding waters.

My wife has us pose
in the shady light,
our backs against thick trunks
rising to the skies.

I read moss on fallen logs,
follow paw prints into brush,
listen to the language of birds,
the bark of another dog.

So wistful, the leisure here
among family and forest,
no subtext or ironies,
ourselves and what is found.

Mountains and Rivers, Earth and Sky

Taking a breath of high air
we know the stillness.
The way is a door,
not narrow but open
wide to all.

And things encountered
on our path are there
to encourage us.
Whatever is, is there
to help us on our way.

Everything without judgment,
imperfect yet clear—
a river we stand in
looking down through its
cool bright surface to
golden rocks our bare feet
rest upon.

Watching Louie Schwartzberg's *Forest* Film

Like the colored leaves in wind,
I drift between wonder and contentment,
time travel through a slow motion and
time-lapse pause of mind. Golden leaves
nestle among rocks and water, then
dissolve to clouds passing overhead like gulls.
We are gliding over and into landscapes
too full to ever hold. A rustle of wind
turns the leaves like hands signaling
a soft breath over all that lives.
A waterfall of music tumbles over rocks
into a pool, where a single leaf drifts down,
lands, sending ripples out into the world, then
floats along within the secret direction
of everything.

The Presence of Absence

for Maj Ragain

I drive back to the old home place
that has been gone for years.
Take the exit off new Route 22
into Florence, Pennsylvania,
a town of a couple thousand,
its crossroads moved west
to the highway now.
Entering town, I pull off
to the north side of the road
where my grandparents lived.

All that is left are trees
and wild underbrush—
locust and sumac and
weeds covering all.
Not even a driveway to mark it.
I sit in my car and look out,
think of my friend whose house
was taken by the waters
of the West Branch dam,
submerged and beyond reach.
Mine taken here by strip mining
then abandoned to wild growth.

I get out, walk around,
search for a place to enter,
a way to sense the old landscape—
taken, changed, robbed
of more than mineral rights.
I must close my eyes to see again
the long front porch, their swing,
the Adirondack chairs that
Grandpa crafted and painted,
the grapevines along the side yard,
Grandma's bright flowers along the back:
rows of gladiolas, irises, beds of petunias,
the old barn back against the trees.

Each year more is taken,
more to remember that can
no longer be seen.
Not even a chimney
to mark a life. I stand
at the edge of the underbrush
and listen long: some birds, crickets,
washed by the rush of traffic nearby.
I reach down for a lone locust shoot,
place it in my water cup
and carry it home.

Lunar Vision

Soft gleam of quarter moon
through deep clouds streaked
across a pale sky—
planetary vision showing
how large our universe. And to the right
a single star beams like another moon
orbiting our own. Wordless voice of
our smallness, our vastness,
our eternal night.

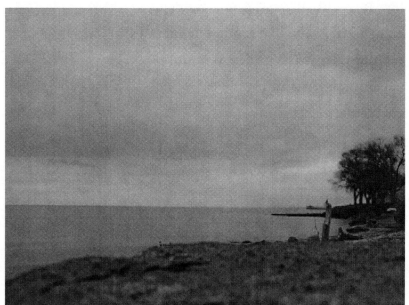
(Photo: Brian Smith)

Family Life

"The family is one of Nature's Masterpieces."
– George Santayana

"If you look deeply into the palm of your hand, you will see your parents and all generations of your ancestors. All of them are alive in this moment. Each is present in your body. You are the continuation of each of these people."
–Thich Nhat Hanh

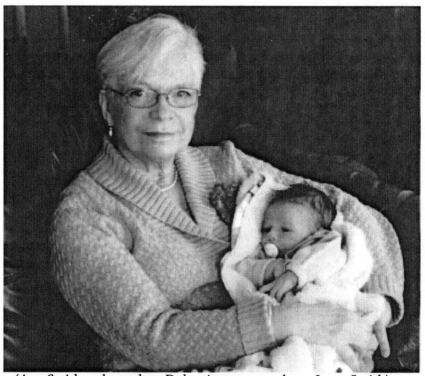
(Ann Smith and grandson Dylan Austerman, photo: Larry Smith)

Finding Ourselves at Brigadoon

Our tour bus heads out of Edinburgh
across Scotland's southern farmlands,
a light rain beating against the windows.

Our driver announces: "The ferry across
to Ireland is down but just for morning,
so we'll take a special side trip."

We are passengers on this voyage
and so settle back to what is next:
cows in a field, old factory towns.

My brother whispers across the seats,
"We're near County Ayr and the village
of Great-Grandfather Cochran."

A continent we've crossed
with our wives, to see this
place of our origins.

The rolling hills, deep green fields,
so like the Alleghenies where he
settled in Pennsylvania.

Ann sleeps at my side as we
glide through countryside,
our guide telling of Scottish ways.

But soon the bus slows
into the town of Alloway,
beautiful homes on quiet streets.

"And who is it that Scotland admires
as poet laureate above the rest?"
our guide asks and waits.

"Why bonny Bobby Burns, the Bard,
my friends; we're at his homelands
here in lovely Alloway."

The bus slows then stops and out the window:
a white stone house with long thatched roof.
"And here is where he lived and wrote."

Beloved poet of Great-Grandfather Cochran,
my grandmother passed along old editions
of Burns' poems to my brother and me.

I rise to take photos from the street
near a bright yellow laburnum tree,
my brother standing by our driver.

Home is written in all of this,
an echo in the heart here,
brought up close before our eyes.

And none so dear and beautiful
as the bridge at Brigadoon, near
the cemetery where Burns' parents lie.

I stand out on the roadway
above the river Doon, camera
pressed to my cheek and eye.

Sheep lie resting on the river bank,
near the stone bridge arcing perfect
across a quiet hillside.

Plants of deep purple and green
grow strong around the grey stone,
the river's stillness deeper than sleep.

My breath quiets and slows:
to find self so far away,
to have touched and known.

Nairn, Scotland

for my mother, Jean

Lying in bed in far north country,
a soft morning light comes on,
and beneath our hotel window
a scent of golden laburnum
joins the songs of new birds.
My wife sleeps secure in blanket and pillows,
while a distant rush of waves
meets the muted cries of gulls.

Away from the roar and rush of Glasgow,
I welcome the slow easy movement
of light into our room—I sleep, I wake,
I sleep to wake and remember…
My Scots-Irish mother quick with wit and caring
rocking me with soft tunes on her sweet breath:
"If a body meet a body, comin' thro' the rye…
If a body kiss a body, need a body cry?" Or
"Did you ever see a laddie, a laddie, a laddie?
Did you ever see a laddie, go this way and that…"
And I close my eyes to hear again,
"Go to sleep my bonnie laddie, Go to sleep my lad…"
Fresh tears for old songs; sweet refrains
echo softly of things long past.

Saturday Mornings 1950s

When Dad would hand over that dollar allowance
to our eager hands after we'd scrubbed the porch
or taken the trash to the end of the yard,
we would grin with satisfaction.
Allowing an hour to pass, I would
head downtown on my bike,
letting her coast down the steep hill,
holding the break pedal steady,
arriving at last on Commercial Street.

I would park it outside Western Auto,
and browse the store for tools and parts,
maybe pick up a new reflector
for my old bike. Then I'd go next door
to the newsstand and scan the comics
for a something new from Plastic Man.
With the quarter that was left,
I'd go over to Islays for a sky cone
of orange sherbet. Maybe sit outside
on the steps and watch people pass,
a neighbor, a friend, a pretty girl from school.
The cone licked away, I would ride
slowly along the sidewalk, past
butcher shop and bakery,

stop at Goodfriends to watch the
new television playing in the window.

Then I would stand at the foot of St. Clair,
and face the long steep hill to home.
Without gears, there was no way to ride her,
and so I would take the handle grips
firm in my hands, lean into her, and
take the hill a step at a time, pushing along,
catching breath at the corners.
At times I'd ride across one street,
but always come to the hill again
at the other side, our way of life.
Finally I would lean my bike
against our front porch and enter
home at last.

Sunday Mornings

While my father shaved, then put on his tie,
we kids wrestled into our clothes:
white shirts for boys, print dresses for girls
that Mom had laid out the night before.
As we gathered at kitchen counter
for cold bowls of cereal and toast,
Mom lay safe asleep upstairs.
We would not see her again till we
returned from Sunday school and church.
I forget who brushed the girls' hair,
but I like seeing my father at the task
his big hands guiding the brush through soft hair,
his handing us the shoe brush for one more swipe.

And we would walk the two blocks to church,
the Smith tribe minus one. And yet
somehow we never resented Mom's absence
because Father never did, and we all knew
how she had earned a break during the week.
Two hours later we would burst through the door
to warm cinnamon rolls and her smiling face.

Days-Off

My father always mixed his cereals,
pouring Cheerio circles onto a
pile of dry Wheaties, dropping
puffed wheat onto puffed rice,
then dumping milk over it all and
mixing it with a large spoon.
Why he did this I'm not sure—
to bring some color to his worker's life?
His day laid out before him like the rails
his train and crew would work upon.

His only cooking was Saturday breakfasts,
French toast squares lined with
strips of salty bacon.
Mom would sleep in, come down
in time to make us wash the dishes,
put the pans away. Dad would disappear
down the steps to the basement
work on a motor or grab his toolbox
and head out to Bill's place or
over to Uncle Ray's garage.
Mom would yell down at him
a list of things that needed
done "right here at home!"
But he'd be already gone into his day.

The summer I worked the mill with him
breathing in the grit and sweat, the long
waiting to punch the clock, I came to know
a measure of his pain, the arc of his caring.

Ferrying

The ferry downriver
goes across every hour,
loaded with river folks,
a few cars, a bicycle or two.
It has been making the crossing
for decades now through seasons.

When I close my eyes, I dream
my father holding a lantern
leaning into the wind
as I watch him in a silence
deep as those waters.

And we glide forward into night
till we strike something hard,
and I wake into the moment
standing on leeward shore
staring across the dark river.

There is so much we could have
said to each other. The silence
now as palpable and smooth
as these waters.

Our last touch, his soft hair,
cold hands, yet in memory alive
and warm as his voice:

Bring that lumber in here, will you?
Now lay them straight, over there.
Here let me show you, son.

Dad, I've met a girl to be my wife
We're going to have a child.

Tell your mother. We'll celebrate.

Dad, we're moving up north for jobs.
I start teaching there in the fall.
We ask your blessing.

You always have it, son.

Our bodies are long rivers
holding birth and death
together, impermanent.

Sunday Drive North of Brilliant, 1948

Just north of town on old Ohio Route 7,
we would slow down for the underpass,
a brief, narrow tunnel dug beneath
the heavy load of railroad tracks.
Which came first the road or the tracks?
It didn't matter, as both lay along the path
of the wide Ohio and those lush green hills.

Our car would be the gray Plymouth
which my uncle sold to my Dad, who drove
beside Mother with baby Janis on her lap,
and on the back seat, brother David and I.
The road would be rough, a ledge really
carved into the bottom of those slanted hills.

As we drove they would begin to sing
the old tunes, but as we neared the underpass
Mom and Dad would stop their singing, like a
radio whose dial was suddenly turned to Off.
For there at the low curve where the road
narrowed would be two boys, one watching
each way and together motioning to us
to come on or to stop.

And their dirty faces
and their eager eyes as we passed, speechless
yet asking, and Dad slowing while Mom dug down
into her purse, then cast out a few pennies
that would land on the ground near their feet.
And the boys would smile and gather up the coins,
probably brothers and only a few years
older than David and I.

For miles as
telephone poles and lines slid by
against a summer sky, I would
sit back and wonder just how we
two boys might apply for their jobs.

Breaking Open

That yellow sweater I wore in the sixth grade
was too pale for a boy in a mill town,
but I was on the edge of innocence then,
still trying to please everyone.

Yes, my mother said I looked good in it,
and my father and brother didn't complain,
but it was a pale yellow like the blonde hair
of Shirley Mae walking before me
down the blind streets of my dreams.

I played hard at gym that day,
taking a quick shower to make it to band
where Shirley and I played cornet.
We were both first chair, both
pressing our lips to the mouth piece.

That Saturday was a birthday party
at Patrick's, down by the tracks.
His mother and aunt smoked in the kitchen
while we played spin the bottle, then post office,
our first kissing games. I was wearing the
yellow sweater when Shirley followed me
into the room. We stood a long while in the
pressing heat of our bodies, then leaned forward

to touch our lips. Just like that I fell though
to a sweetness I would never forget. After she left,
I smelled the odor of my own sweat.

Reunion at Cross Creek

for David

Walking the hills back home
to the near side of the river,
a light snow in morning sun.

Back at the house, people will be rising
taking hot showers, combing hair,
eggs turned to suns on plates.

I have gone out to a place where
we once fished along a creek.
The whisper of traffic overhead
on the bridge near railroad tracks.

A dozen starlings
rooting among leaves
on the frozen bank.

I close my eyes, and my brother
appears on the other side
bending to light a fire.

"Let's see what's biting here," he says.
"We'll go home in a little while."

I sit on a log counting breaths and
disappearing in the sunny dawn.

Convergence–Brothers

My brother and his wife drive up
for lunch and a visit.
For years he and I slept
in the same room, falling asleep
to his clock radio.

Wordless in morning light
we dressed for school.
Dad gone to work already,
Mother sleeping still,
then sisters rising with her
to bowls of kitchen cereal.

Dave would head out
before me with his friends,
and I would wait for mine.
Our paths crossing
in a silence understood.

Wounded Hearts

I.

My father died 200 miles away—
at the age of 65, and I ,now 70,
still carry the weight of that loss.
No time then to say the things
we never spoke aloud. No time
to share his pain or ease his passing.
200 miles which we drove to
be with my mother, sisters, brother,
to hear Mom tell of his arriving home
taking cookies in his hand, saying
"I'm going upstairs to lie down."
Her finding him there on the bed,
touching him to be sure.

And me 200 miles away at a meeting—
my wife come to call me out, saying
"Your father…he's gone," there on the stairs,
my cry of anguish rising from my chest, echoing,

her holding me close.

II.

Driving us back home through
thoughts of him: images of
his shoulders and arms, his hands

working a hammer or drill,
his face open, softly strong—
all being pulled from me.
"He's gone," she said but knew
I'd find him again somehow.

The arrangements, the gatherings,
stories being told by old friends,
talks with my bother and sisters.
Mom holding it all in, me aching to be free.
The standing together at the grave
in morning light, my uncle's face of tears.

III.
It was summer and so others went home
while I stayed on to help.
And so began the cleaning up,
the putting away, the signing of papers,
driving Mom in the car, both of us
alone with him in our way.
Waking in their house early in silence,
eating breakfast where he had been.
Mom's wanting things done
and gone, my still holding on to all.
Each act a sign of his loss, sharp betrayal
for all the times not there for him.
The giving away of his tools and clothes—

my cousin and I hauling out boxes

from the basement to the town dump,

throwing them there on the fire.

Mom not wanting to hear of it,

and so at night I would call Ann,

my safe lifeline to other family.

IV.

Then after a week, my sister came

to watch over Mom, and so I

was released, to make the drive home.

200 miles to think and feel, no

longer divided, tears coming as I drove,

rounding Tappan Lake, our old fishing hole.

And then halfway home, nearing Canton,

the sun resting into the hills,

I took a long breath and felt him—there

with me in the car. He was there

in the sky, the road, the tires,

the air we were passing through. He was

everywhere like God and would remain

with me all the days of my life and beyond.

The Storyteller's Story

for Sue

Did she choose to be a storyteller
or did storytelling choose her?
I'm the only one who wonders this still;
for all the others it is just who she was,
Sue, the family storyteller. As a young girl
helping her mother with dishes and food,
she'd serve a dessert of family tales
holding all round the kitchen table,
looking all deep in their eyes, her
face twisting with the events, her
hands slapping the table, her
voice rising and falling off
as she danced the telling
into their hearts and minds.

As she grew older, married with children,
the telling remained, the same stories
timed like the meals she served.
A word, a look, a question
would bring them on. No matter
what she was doing, she'd stop,
turn back the clock to the first telling.
Her eyes would come alive,
her voice fill with feeling.

A hundred times, yet she could not
escape their saying, though some folks
drifted from kitchen to living room.
She noticed, but continued the telling
with the lessons held inside each tale—
the storyteller's duty.

And I, the son-in-law, sat and watched
in awe without interruption.
Once alone together, I called her
a *raconteur* and she turned on me like a cat.
"No," I said, "I only wish
I could write stories like yours."
She smiled and sighed, "But, oh,
if I could only write them down, I
wouldn't have to keep telling them."

When she was 86, she fell twice
and broke each hip, and with
that loss, she felt the bite of age
into her memory cells. Each year,
each month, she remembered less.
At first the closest things, the pan
left on the stove, what she had just started,
how to drive home from town.
And then the longer things went, like
when we last saw her, where they once lived,

the names of her brothers and sisters.
We prompted her, enabling her
to go on, because we couldn't bear
losing her. But so she went
into the darkness of dementia, and soon
we moved her into nursing care,
a place where she sat in wheelchair
and watched the sun go up and down.
Family would visit, lean toward her
waiting for her stories to come pouring out,
prompting her with all they still held
of her telling…words, names, events.
But no stories came from her lips,
no tales came to those eyes.
And when she could barely talk, just
stare at us as strangers, she once
asked my wife: "And how is your mother?"

Freed of her stories, she has left us
to tell them to ourselves.

Flowers

We are shopping for flowers
to take to my old aunt Mary
when my wife remembers her
grandmother hanging geraniums
by their roots in the cellar.
"'Putting them to sleep,' she called it,
then planting them again next spring,"
Ann says as we stroll past
pots of tulips, yellow and blue.

Back in our hometown,
we drive a purple hyacinth
on our back seat up the hill
to her yellow brick house.
We have not seen her in a year
and fear the weathering of age.
At the door, she looks fine
in a red blouse and well coiffed hair.
Her arms are thin as the narrow
shafts of bamboo plants, her voice
is weak as the forsythia blooms
outside in the wind. We touch
lightly, both afraid she will break.

She takes the flowers, smiles,

and asks us in. "The cleaning girl
was here this morning," she says,
"You're in luck," and sits on her
navy blue couch. Ann places
the hyacinth on the glass table-top
asks loudly, "How are you doing?"
She turns like a crane in water,
"Oh…I'm well enough," she says,
"What can we expect at this age?"

We laugh a moment and I feel relief
that she is still here, remember
the aunt of vacation trips, her fast driving,
whispering things to my mother, her hands
banging piano keys, beating me at cards,
her gray head singing in the choir.
Inside this frail body of hers
she lives on. I smile and then she speaks,
"The cleaning girl was here this

morning. You're in luck."

For Giving

for Grandma Ferroni

She moves about her kitchen
like a ship captain at sea
gliding from one task to another
lifting pans, stirring sauce,
dropping eggs into table flour
to mold into her daily bread
shared with neighbors.

She pauses to make tea,
sits with her rosary and prayers.
Outside, the distant roar
of mill yard reminds her of him,
gone now ten years. At the funeral
when her older sister Flora said,
"You think it's bad now, huh?
Well, I tell you, it only gets worse,"
her daughter had wanted to spit back,
yet she had only smiled through tears,
then squeezed Flora's hand and
whispered, "Say a prayer for me."

"God bless them," she would say
to all news of family and neighbors.
All gossip and criticism would
melt before her forgiveness,

her soft hands, her serving of
cookies and tea, even to children
seated around kitchen table.

The young girl who crossed the ocean
to America still lives inside her.
At times she might tell the story
of the leaking ship and her
finding a wooden cross come
floating up to her bunk.
"Have faith," she would say
taking your hand in hers. And her
"Bless them" would open you
to new lands.

Holding On

I wake in the night
to a sound and then
my lost mother's voice
speaking just my name.

Gone now twenty years
it carries comfort and concern
calling me back and beyond.
I lie back then rise to walk
out to 3 a. m. darkness.

All families must struggle
shed tears of joy and sadness
face the mistakes and losses
that are our lives.

"Keep close," she used to say
hugging me at the door...
"Don't forget your old mother,"
She would smile and pat my arm.

I hold her close now
in my mind and heart
as I do my children,
my wife and self.

Welcoming

for Ann

I lie in bed as morning light comes on
and listen to my wife's gentle breathing,
like waves coming in and out upon the shore.
We have crossed many days, many years together.

I slide my body next to her softness, breathe in
her warmth, the flower smell of her hair.
She rests deeply here from all of her caring.
Soon I will rise and make our coffee,
greet her waking face with a kiss.

The Dance...

Written to music of Lou Young
for Laura and Suzanne

The dance begins. Young ballerinas in the dancing hall—
pirouette, bend, extend their arms like lovely swans.
 I sit among the parents watching through glass,
my mind quiet at last—here only to watch
and receive these gifts of measure.
We are one in this time and space, this big room,
this life where time falls away…falls away, falls away.
"How to tell the dancer from the dance?"

The girls dressing afterwards laugh softly.
I look into the eyes of my daughter and wonder
at the miracle of her birth—my child—
come dancing into my heart.

Walking the Lake Together

for Laura

She is 47 now, woman-wife-mother and
daughter still, two thousand miles away.

We follow the path among tall trees,
sweet scent of Cedar and Spruce.
"Your Walden Pond," I say, and she laughs
that young girl laugh of hers.

She stops to point out the floating reeds
"like a line drawing" along the shore.
I smile and take a photograph.

We cross a stone bridge, walk out a quiet pier,
look down through calm clear water.

She takes my picture with lake.
I take hers with trees.

She means so much to me
I cannot speak, and so we walk
the silent shoreline together.

Lessons

for Brian

Walking through a dark woods
past brush and fallen logs
our dogs find the way.

I tell my son, "We are lost."
"No," he says, "What's lost is home."

*   *   *

We tread through bush and bramble
at times carrying our pups
over puddles and muck.
At first I lead the way,
and then I follow him.

A Working Mom

for Suzanne

Mother of three, like her mom,
our daughter dresses each child,
tries to get some breakfast
into them and herself.
Always looking sharp, she moves
with efficiency, lays out the schedule,
packs each off to school
before heading to the V.A.
Listening there as at home,
perhaps directing someone
away from harm, touching
old men and her children
with care. Between the moments
of concern, she catches breath,
does yoga beside her desk.
Driving home she calls her Joe
then chats with her mother.
Evening dishes served and cleaned
children storied into bed,
she and Joe nestle on the couch
talk of their day before
falling fast asleep.

Bellingham Breakfast

for Rosa

Sitting in the Old Town Café
we wait our eggs,
as a few white clouds
float over Lummi Island.

My granddaughter plays
with her sausage. Her eyes
are brown marbles, gems really,
as she almost smiles.
She is fourteen and hungry
for experience, boys, romance,
that first kiss.

She writes it all in notebooks,
stories of others living her
dreams and nightmares.
She thinks no one likes her.
I stare at her hands, fingers long and
fine around her water glass.

My wife and daughter
sip tea, grandson plays
in the corner. Then Laura says,
"Oh, I didn't tell you.

Rosa has a part in school play."
Even Rosa smiles at this,
bubbles with stories.

And I am remembering fourteen
so much of time spent waiting
for moments like this when
life is a meal to be eaten.

Growing into Himself

I am a grain of rice.

I am a tree in the wind.

I am a day to night cycle.

I am a shard of glass slowly being curved.

I am a flickering candle.

I am a piece of thread holding a quilt.

I am a black cat in the night.

I am a new invention finding perfection.

I am what I am. That is what I am.

-Rustle Frost (age 9)

These words come to us in Ohio

from our West Coast grandson

who has always danced his life forward.

Agile in words and action with tousled hair,

he beckons with his big trusting eyes.

Part athlete, magician, comedian,

bouncer on trampoline, he does flips

into our hearts.

Born at home before the midwife

could arrive, his mother and father

brought him safe into this world

and into our lives.

He has always surprised with

his father's wit, his mother's gentleness.

He is that rice grain, that candle, cat, and thread,

that tree growing into himself.

Working Together

Today we dig in the yard,
planting lights instead of flowers
along the edge of porch.
Three grandkids and I,
my son's children
themselves lights in darkness.
Adam digs on ahead, Alex
runs for tools, and Zoe
plays on the steps in sun,
while I work the wiring.

Lake wind is crisp for March,
yet winters' leaves must be raked
from between the bushes.
I follow Adam's steady trench
planting wire, my hands
reaching down into dark earth
broken open for me.
As we pause to test, while Zoe
buzzes about each of us.
At three everything's a wonder;
as for me, almost seventy,
this working together
at bringing light
sets life free.

A Story of War

for Adam

My grandson and I visit the history museum.
He is six and always asking, so we
tour the cases, a war for each one,
beginning with 1812, fought off-shore on Lake Erie.
But what has drawn him into history's web
is the Civil War, book images of men
in a field wielding swords and bayonets
and long rifles—"How many inches, Grandpa?"

I am a pacifist, a veteran of no wars,
yet I walk with him and his questions.

Two days ago we strolled the Confederate Cemetery
on Johnson's Island, where men locked up men
and buried those who could not survive.
And what is left are head stones and small Rebel flags,
a tall statue of one with his long gun—
put up by the Daughters of the Confederacy.

A young boy and an old man among headstones,
I try to explain to him and myself
the reasons for that war and others.
And he looks up at me in mid-sentence, in that
field of graves and says, "Grandpa, I would not

risk my life to kill another person"—That simple
and true to his own innocence. I tell him

I honor their bravery but not their killing.
"Right," he says, and we let that moment stand
as our being together on a battleground.

We trade the museum for lunch in a diner.
Over milkshakes and burgers, he says,
"Grandpa, I love the war." And I, "You do?"
"Not the killing. Not that, but your stories
of the battlefields." I somehow know
and let it stand, a truth between us.

Silent on the long drive home,
I turn to say, "I love you, Adam.
I am not going to die for a long time."
And he answers back, "Never."

Fishing the Lake

What we came for, and what arrives.
My grandson and I walk out the pier
all the way to the lighthouse,
carrying our fishing poles and gear
navigating the huge boulders
that drop off into a deep lake.
If he falls in, I will follow
unable to live with his loss.

I bring a bucket of shiners
that we will put back into the lake
two by two, hoping against wind
to draw out a perch or bass,
perhaps a great walleye
to celebrate the day together
in the sun and wind.

The steady hoot of the lighthouse,
the waves washing up on the rocks,
the old guy who shows him
how to bring it in without a snag.
We calculate then cast out,
letting go the line, learning to
sit and wait again and again.
What we came for, and what arrives.

Sharing the Night

He lies here beside me, my grandson,
moaning softly into the night,
his younger brother a bed away
asleep by my wife. And I
do not know how to console him
or ease his unspoken pain.

I stroke his tight muscled back,
his tender arms. And finally
I reach across my own
unloveableness to hold him,
whisper softly, "You're okay, hon.
We love you." Words my father
could not say, words I forced out
for my own son, his father.

How to read a young boy's pain or need.

I rise to get him a drink, cover
his bare legs, then lie back,
feel his breathing in and out,
close my eyes again, as together
we move softly into the night.

The Gift

for Adam

"Write a poem about this, Grandpa,"
he says as we stand together
in the rainy shelter-house watching
townsfolk stand in line as the son
signs his books at a table,
the father selling them at this side.

"Write a poem about this," Adam says again.
"I know you will." I smile
at my own love for him,
so young and wise, who sees
a light in me still, though the
world so often grows dim.

Sitting alone as dawn comes on,
I remember and I write.

Another Home Burial

for Alex

It begins with a dead bird.
No, with a bird house just made
by my grandson and me.
Alex is almost four and
curious as the wind.
When we find a place to hang it,
we discover an old one nearby.

"But how do the birds get in,"
he asks. Without looking
I say, "Through the hole,"
but he is right, the hole is closed,
stuffed with nesting I suppose.
I take it down and he hands me a stick.
But no, what's stuffed in the hole
is a dead bird—twisted legs and wing.
I pull out the corpse, all dry bones and feathers.

Alex drinks all this in—fear and fascination
mixed with a sly smile of adventure.
I tell him we must bury it.
"Why"" he asks as I retrieve a shovel.
Why? I ask myself. "It's what we do
when something dies," I say

and continue the ancient rite.
He watches, then helps me
plant the tiny body, then
we cover all with grass.

Back in the garage we wash our hands
again and again, wiping away
all trace of disease and death.
His puzzled look draws my words:
"Remember when your lizards died—
you and Adam buried them." He nods.
"And our dog Bear. When the vet
put him to sleep, We buried him."
"Where?" he wants to know.
"In the woods," I say, kneeling down.
"I took him there and dug a hole,
and laid him down, then covered him
with dirt and leaves..."
His face is a bowl of silence.

We put away our tools. It's time
to pick up his brother. On the way
he says, "You put Bear in a hole
and buried him"—half in question.
"Yes," I say, and he: "Don't ever
do that again!" I pause at this,
turn round to mirror his confusion.

He looks straight into my eyes.
Both of us caught in that half understanding—
answers and questions awakened.

We pick up his brother whose chatter
silences Alex. But when we get home
he runs in to Grandma, he gasps, "Grandpa
put Bear in a hole!" Ann stares at me.
I nod. She thinks it through. "Yes,
he did do that." "But where?" he insists.
"Why, honey?" she kneels to ask.
"Because," he says half out of breath,
"I want to go there and dig him up."

Picking Up Alex

I stand with the young mothers
outside the school doors at 3:25,
waiting for the children to be released.
My little dog barks at each,
then sits quiet at my feet.
Suddenly the door opens
and a woman calls out their names,
cattle released at the gate.
Alex comes running to me,
"Grandpa," he shouts, throws his arms
around my legs. I pat his back,
and take his school bag, hand him
a fruit treat, then the leash to Pokey
who nuzzles at his feet.
"How was school," I ask, and
he again says, "Good."

We walk together across and
up the street to our house, where
Ann has made an afterschool treat.
He hugs her too, then sits to eat.
Here he tells a story, sometimes true,
of what went on at school or home.
Once he told us he woke up late, his

dad was gone, and so he walked

two miles to school. "No!" we said.

"Yes, and it was cold crossing that bridge."

We called to ask. A storyteller,

he holds the truth like coins,

till he wants to spend them.

He rises to help me make afternoon coffee,

measures and pours in the water.

"What are we doing today?" he asks,

and I say "Flying a plane across to Canada."

He questions my face, says, "No, we are not."

I laugh, say, "Let's go feed the birds."

He takes the seed pitcher from my hand,

pours it in the way I do. "Good job,"

I say and bend to kiss his red hair.

"You're weird," he says and walks away,

following his older brother's path into age.

Later he will sit and eat with us,

carry meat and salad with his fork.

Then he'll clear the table and disappear,

till we find him on the couch, fast asleep

from his day's work.

Breathing New Life into It

for Maya

Our granddaughter plays with the manger scene,
moving the animals and shepherds and kings
about the buffet, talking softly with them.

MayA takes up baby Jesus, manger and all,
and holds him to her breast.

And then everyone moves out.
Kings and shepherd, cow and sheep,
circle the golden tree on the
Christmas table cloth, now
talking with each other.

Only the donkey rests inside, Joseph kneeling to him.

Then all are quiet as she lifts baby Jesus up
to the rooftop where he kneels to
kiss the lone angel hanging there.

The Bedtime Story

> for Maya

At bedtime, we divide the granddaughters.
Ann is taking 4 year old Alyssa, and I'll
tuck in 7 year old Maya.
Stories will be required for both.
Maya has it all planned, and in pink pajamas
retrieves a journal from her bedroom closet.
"These are **my** stories," she whispers loud
and climbs in bed beside me.
Her handwriting and line drawings
are spread across the pages. Her spelling
is as original as her characters.
The first is of a rude bunny who must
learn to say she's sorry to friends.
And then she tells me that four boys
in her class have crushes on her,
and she on only one, Zach. I smile
and tell her the story of my first kiss.
"You mean not from your mother or dad?"
"Yes," I say, "My first kiss from a girl."
She giggles at this and waits,
"I was in fourth grade…let's see, I'd be
9 years old then, as old as some of the girls
and boys in your piano recital today."
She nods. "I was at a birthday party,

and we played kissing games...can you believe it...
Spin the Bottle, did you ever hear of that?"
Her giggles have already become ripples.
 "Really?" she asks, "Yes," I nod.
"and we were only fourth graders."
"Tell what happened," she instructs. "Did you
have to kiss a girl?" "Well, yes, I did," I say,
"a cute blonde girl named Shirley Mae."
"How, how did you do it?" she wants to know.
I try to recall... "Well, it was very lightly, like this,"
and I make a short kiss in the air. Sweet giggles again,
and I ask, "Have you ever kissed a boy?" Her eyes
get big as she smiles but shakes her head no.
She is such a sweet girl, and I wonder if I'm going
too far with this talk of kissing. She'll tell her mother,
my daughter, and I'll surely hear of it. But then,
she says, "Wait, I have another story," and she turns
to the back of the book. "This is secret," she whispers.
We come to two snowmen on separate pages.
"He's a snow boy...and she's a snow girl,"
silly laughter again. "I see," I say.
 "We don't need words," she says, "I'll tell you
their story," and she begins. "You see, he asks this snow girl
if she likes him, and she tells him 'No.'"
"Ah..." I let on. "Wait," she says, "it's just begun."
The pages flip to show our dejected snow boy
with another snow girl, and soon the first snow girl

begins to notice. Trouble is brewing, but then

a new snow boy appears and draws attention

from snow girl #2…They go off, and now snow girl #1

turns to our snow boy and says, "Yes, I do like you."

Maya looks over at me, and I nod. "Wait," she smiles

and turns to the last page…two snow people kissing.

We laugh together…and I notice something.

"What are those things on the ground?"

"Guess, Grandpa," she demands…and when I give up,

she tells me, "Those are their noses.

They had to take them off to kiss."

Blossomings

for Zoe Miranda and Alyssa Ann

As I gaze into the faces
of our new granddaughters
bright eyes and gentle smiles
beckoning my heart to trust,
I wonder just how long
I'll be responsible to them.
As long as I am able.

Like their brothers and sisters
they have changed their parents' lives
forever. Their tiny fingers
now reach out like roots
into the loose turf of my life
holding me together, giving me
safe ground to dream for them:
cousins like sisters,
one day walking together
to the beach, blowing out candles
on each other's cakes,
spinning around in fine dresses,
their lovely faces saying *Yes,*
me too in your life.

The Lives of the Ain'ts

Here's to those who refuse the status quo
who make it new again and again
rebelling out of love not hate
creating fresh paths
and bidding us do the same
who awaken a self
guided only by the heart's truth
in the now presence

To kids who roll their eyes at teacher commands
asking questions in the face of silence
who cross the lines they believe are wrong
and to parents who let children run free
To those who grow beards and dreadlocks
who shave their heads, dye hair pink or red

To artists who touch us wisely
jazzmen playing beyond any score
finding notes and rhythms that
open outward to light
To dancers turning inside and out
caught in the music of love
and to writers pushing and pulling us
over the edge to the sea

No count of martyrdom here
none of them asking for pay
or recognition or advancement
Each in tune with a vision
of giving and living free
in the moment and for all time.

The Time-Out

for Alyssa

I enter the time-out zone of my bedroom
where granddaughter Alyssa lies across the bed.
"I'm getting a time-out," she confesses,
and I say, "I know," as I lie down beside her.
She is almost five and I almost seventy,
but this really doesn't matter. I ask,
"Is it okay that I lie down here?"
She nods and comes closer to share my pillow.
Her little voice and face show no signs of
regret for throwing the Play-Doh toys
or not saying she was sorry.
But I have not come to punish.

We breathe together for a little while,
and I begin to tell her a story.
I am a boy of five joining the fight
with the new neighbor kids, chasing them
home with small rocks when I let one go
and it flies quick into the front window
of their house where my family used to live.
Crack—and *smash* goes the glass,
and I stare at the kid my age, as both of us
shudder in the crash. "You're in big trouble,"
he says, and I answer, "I hate you."

My big brother shakes his head
as I turn and begin running my way home
leaving one fear for another.

Guilt tastes like metal in my mouth as I
tell my mother. "Oh, my god!" she screams,
"Not that big front window?"
My granddaughter is held in stillness.
"Was it?" she asks, "The big window?"
"Yes," I confess to her as to my mother.
Mom frowned; my granddaughter grins.
And I tell her how my mother comes out of
her gasp to say, "Go, you. Sit in the front room
and wait for your father to come home.
You must tell him," and she walks away.
I do as she asks and sit as a prisoner of my guilt.
An hour later when my father comes home
from the mill, I look up into his face.
"What's the story?" he asks, sensing something.
"I did something bad," I tell him. "I broke a window
by throwing a rock at the Kennedy's house."
"Oh my god! Not the big front window?"
I nod again, hang my head waiting to be struck
by a man who has never struck me.
There is only silence as he thinks, then finally:
"Boy," he says, "Come with me." And I rise.
"We're going up there for you to tell them

you are sorry." As we walk up the hill,
I almost wish he had paddled me
and wiped the slate clean.
Alyssa stares right into my face.
"I was afraid he wouldn't love me," I say,
and her eyes get big as she swallows.
"And did you say it, that you were sorry?"
she needs to know. "Yes, I did," I tell her,
"and I was sorry for everyone…for them,
their old house, for my dad and mom, and for myself."
She lies there silent and then she asks,
"And did they still love you?"
I hadn't thought of this.
"Oh, yes, they did. My father said to me
as we walked home, 'Listen, son, what you
did was surely wrong, you know that.
And somehow you'll help pay for it
by helping me install the new glass.'
But then he stroked my arm, the one
which had thrown the rock, and told me,
'But you are not bad, and you know too
that we still love you.'"
Alyssa breathes out a sigh with this.
We lie there quiet for a few minutes
just breathing and thinking together
when finally she turns to me to say,
"Grandpa. Tell me another story."

This story doesn't end here, for an hour later,

after we two have gathered up Play-Doh toys

and she has told Grandma she is sorry,

I tell her, "You know we love you still."

She looks back at me and whispers

just loud enough for me to hear,

"And your father…"

"Yes?" I lean toward her.

"He loves you too."

Beach Chase

I in my ball cap and bare feet
take off chasing grandson Dylan
in his diaper and cap down the beach.
He wobbles slightly yet runs way ahead
leaving baby footprints in the wet sand.
An older couple watching the chase,
calls out, "How old is he?" as though
they want to place a bet.
I yell, "Eighteen months," but must
increase my pace. He's too near the edge
and could dart off into lake waters.

When I catch and lift him into the air,
he gives off a high giggle and smiles
into my worried face which smiles back
as I hug his bare body to my chest.
His mother standing at our blanket
watches her father and son
embrace on the beach.
I bend to set him down and he
takes off again, this time
towards her and home.

Touching Bugs

for Dylan

My grandson and I water flowers
in our back yard. Walking at 18 months
he carries the watering pail.
Each time he catches on more,
smiles and crouches down
next to the flowers as his water
pours over them.

Midway through he loses attention
and turns to touch the tiny ant
moving across the pavers,
a thing so small I hadn't seen it.
He's closer to the ground, yes,
but also he's more open to all
as part of his world.

I call him my Zen teacher
even when he pushes the ant
into its next life.

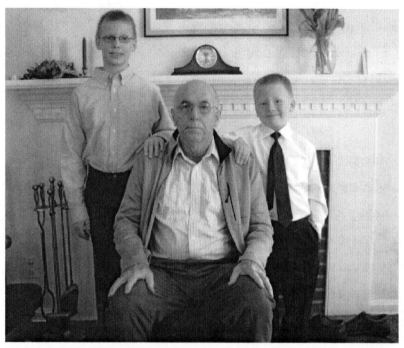

Larry with grandsons Adam and Alex, 2012, photo: Brian Smith

The Bill Poems

So Live

So live life that upon your leaving:

whether recognized or not, (it should not matter)

the world will be a better place

because you lived.

-William C. Wright from *A Life in Poems*

[William C. Wright (Bill, 1914-2012) was a friend to all. He served in WW II and as a union organizer, peace and justice activist, humanitarian, and lover of nature and his good wife Chris. During the last years of his life my wife and I cared for Bill, and it proved to be not a burden but a blessing.]

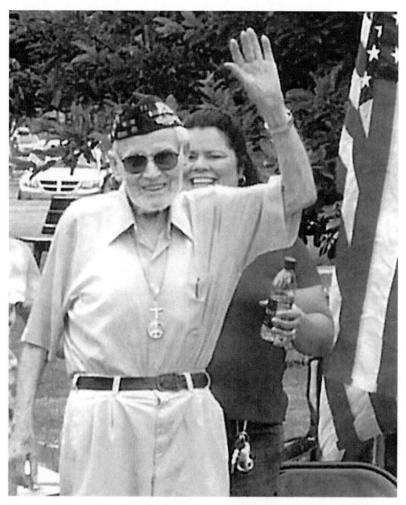

Bill Wright at July 4th, 2009 gathering in Sandusky wearing his
Veterans for Peace cap, photo: Larry Smith

Our Bill of Rights

> for Bill Wright on his 90th birthday

Bill grew up on the Wright farm
down in Huron County, Ohio with
brothers Vernon and Paul, and sweet sister Illene.
Bill milked cows for the family dairy—
did early morning deliveries with his father
who talked of justice and freedom, and
taught him the sharing of milk with those in need,
as Bill would come to do for the WIC program.

Bill earned his place during high school as a boxer,
then as a bass player in Ohio Vaudeville.
With others he marched for social security,
fair wages, racial equality, a safe workplace.
It became his way of life:
machinist, electrical worker, handyman,
organizer in the 30s, 40s, 50s, and beyond.
He walked the picket lines,
took a beating but held his ground,
asking the hard questions of us all.

After the war, Bill and his beloved Chris
built a house of peace along the lake
where animals, water, land and sky
welcomed the world. Forty years

they sang and danced together
as lovers and friends to us all.

Bill is still with us, working for justice—
standing in the cold and rain
around a picket barrel fire,
telling stories to the young
of working people and their dreams,
writing poems of family and Nature,
turning truths to songs for us all.

We love you, Bill, for
being true to your beliefs,
to what you feel and
who you are.

Working with Bill: Against the Sighing of Trees

Bill is ninety-three this year,
something I tell his bankers
and lawyers while tending his affairs.
"Bill is ninety-three and growing frail"—
words that speaks of value
and the sighing of trees.

In his house he has saved papers
and clippings by the decades,
stored in folders and a hundred
boxes and filing drawers.
We classify by his interests and concerns:
social justice, racism, education,
world affairs, the history of Russia and Cuba,
Erie and Huron Counties.
I ask about some and his voice is soft
but insistent like lake wind.

Lining the shelves are books
of archeology, art, Nature, Indian lore,
American history, and poetry.
"I always thought I would use these,"
he sighs, "to write on someday, but now..."
and he turns up the palms of his thin hands
in question or doubt or release.

We keep filing to make space,
gathering his own poems, my taking
the photos to his hands, each one
a time and place, a story he tells
while I stack the boxes:
how he met his fair wife Chris
while passing petitions for the Scottsboro Boys,
their love letters during World War II,
tales of union organizing across Ohio,
their singing "Joe Hill" in Black churches,
she talking with the women in kitchens,
he gathering the men to strike.

Bill speaks softly of Chris' last days;
her fair haired photos shine in every room.

Sometimes the radio plays symphonies
behind his recalling the family farm,
the dairy business, his brothers and sister,
a mother who wouldn't love him, a father
who did in silence. "My memory
is going," he says, "and I can't get it back."
I have no words to answer this, and so
I gather and sort, finally say, "You've
led a good life, Bill." He nods and smiles,
"I know. I never thought I'd live this long."

And the story could end here,
only it doesn't, as he goes on
teaching me and others to voice
our caring, to build on brother- and
sisterhood. He stands at a doorway now
offering me his hand, his sharp face one
of justice against the wind.

The Promise

My old friend Bill tells me
of how he walks his block
to keep his legs moving.
Only now his face
so thin and frail
speaks of an old pain.
"Young boys," he says,
"are shooting at birds."
Now Bill has known hunting
and battles and war,
yet this needless killing
brings new tears to his eyes.

"I want you to do something."
And I look up in helpless question.
What can anyone do to stop violence?
He takes my hand and says,
"Take some of my money, please,
and buy small bird books
that I can put in their hands."
I pause, look into his so blue eyes,
and then I promise yes.

Going Home

I drive my old friend out to the lake shore
where he used to live. The "Chausse" they call it,
a narrow peninsula strip that leads on to an
amusement park at the edge of Lake Erie.

Almost 95 now, Bill wonders at the new houses,
the sand blown over banks onto the road.
"There must have been a storm," he says,
holding onto his cane. "We had our share of those."
He has forgotten their house number, and so we
watch for the water tower above their frame house.

He and his beloved Chris lived here for five decades.
"She was a wonderful swimmer," he confides.
"I had to work 11-hour days delivering milk,
but we would walk the beach at night."
And I point out a water tower covered with a dark rust.
"Yes, that's it," he whispers, and we pull off
onto a driveway that leads to a bay house.
"Oh!" he exclaims. "It's so different."
I have been to his old place long ago,
a small blue cottage too near the lake's waters.
"They must have raised it, put a basement under it."
He wants to believe it's the same house
risen somehow from past into future.

It is double the size and new, yet I agree, "Yes, they have."
"We always had floods," he tells me. "I worked
11-hour shifts back then, never got round to raising it."

We pull onto a gravel driveway behind a lumber truck.
A worker comes out to ask, "You fellows want something?"
I roll down my window and smile, "This man used to live here."
He grins, "Mr. Wright? Is that you?" and
reaches his calloused hand in to shake Bill's.
"I'm John, the one who bought your place."
Bill cannot hear, yet recognizes the face, reaches
across me to take his hand. "Oh, yes. How are you?"
"I'm great," he smiles, "We love it here.
Would you like to see inside?"

And we pull around to the front door.
When I get out, the lake wind almost knocks me over.
        What will it do to Bill?
Flecks of an April snow blow against our cheeks
as we stand beside the car. Bill totters on a board
placed at the outer threshold of the porch.
We both eye that front step. Too high—he will never
be able to raise his leg or stand alone on the other,
even while I hold him up. "No," he tells me. "I can't."
The other fellow and I could easily lift his 115 pounds,
but then I see—he doesn't want or need to have erased
the life they shared together in that time and place.

We lean together facing the wind.

"We had a garden over there," he tells me.

"Chris and I would sit here and fish,

then we'd watch the sun set into our lake."

The Way Home

Sitting in his favorite diner,
again Bill orders what I order,
eggs and bacon with toast.
He tells me of times
he's been here before.
His food grows cold
while I fill my mouth.

His talking is to hang on
to what mind he has left.
He's slipping and knows it
…hangs on…hangs on.
The waitress takes our plates,
"Still working on yours, hon?"
"Yes," he says and takes another bite
to prove it to her and himself.
He's telling me how he's
tried reading the paper and
can't make sense of it.
Not just the sentences that
seem to run off, but
the world itself gone astray.

The past is secure, he knows it,
holds it somewhere

in the back rooms of his mind.
Old photos of Chris start it
like an old car that he once drove
around the block when young.
He hasn't driven for a decade.
He's tried watching tv and
can't follow it either—
the quick turns, threads lost.
He hates this feeling,
losing his way in the coming dark
just wants to get home, to rest,
to fall into her arms and sleep.

Over Soft Ground

Two days of rain and yet we drive
south together over county roads
to his family's resting plots.
As we drive through town
his memory latches onto
old buildings, railroad tracks, houses:
"Uncle Luke built that place
during the Great Depression
from cement blocks he made…
Chris's father ran a machine shop
in that building over there."
He gives me landmarks for
a town I've only passed through.

As we enter Woodlawn Cemetery
a gather of grackles rise
from the ground to the trees,
finding seed and shelter
wherever they can.
At ninety-four he cannot recall
where the family plots lay,
yet we know a small crypt
stands at the top of a hill,
an oak below rises
above the graves.

Bill reads the names on markers,
finding neighbors and friends,
rocking gently with memories:
"Reverend Garcia, my old teacher…
he married Chris and me…
seems like just yesterday."
And I do not say it was
seventy years ago.

We circle drives, look out
for the Ransom mausoleum.
Names fall from his dry lips.
And then we see it: a
limestone structure on a rise.
I pass slowly, look down a hill
where the oak spreads its arms.
Rain spatters the windshield
as I stop. He reaches for the door.
I say, "Wait, please. Let me
make sure it's the right place."
I tell him this twice, then
step out into the drizzle.

Brown…No…Jones…No…
Always the Smiths…old markers
deep in the ground…There
along the edge one rises:

"Billy Wright…1939-1941,"
his infant son. And there too
rest his father and mother.
I turn, but he is already out
walking towards me with his cane.
I rush to him fearing his fall,
and we walk together through
wet grass, over uneven soil, to
where his family rest in the ground.

Standing in spring rain at dusk where
decades ago Bill spread his wife's ashes
over his baby's grave,
we find his tears.

Taking Bill to the VA

I arrive at Bill's place at 8 a.m.
to take him for his blood test, and
he is already washed and dressed.
Paula has placed signs around
telling him "Do not eat or drink."
"Oh, Larry," he exclaims,
from the lounge chair that he
almost lives in now, "Boy, am I
glad to see you." I smile at
the welcome, say, "Morning, Bill,
we're going for tests at the VA."
"Oh, I forgot," he apologizes.
He forgets everything new now,
clings to old stories to navigate.
His house is a gallery of old photos:
his wife Chris gone 30 years now,
his boy Billy who died at 18 months.
"How old am I?" he asks and ponders.
"96?" he guesses and I nod in this
ritual we play each visit.
"We'll get breakfast," I say
loud enough not to repeat. "Oh, good,
I don't think I've eaten yet."
I help him stand up, hand him one
of the 3 canes we've bought.

"The cheapest is good enough," he said
and says again now, as he did
when we made his funeral plans.
Sitting across the table from a pretty girl
Bill joked, "I'm cheap I guess. But
I'll be gone…just my ashes left behind."
He gazed into her face, smiled, "So nice
to talk with someone so young."

Paula has laid out his heavy coat,
and I hold it behind as he reaches back,
each arm finding its sleeve. "It's cold," I say.
"What?" he asks. "It's cold outside," I say.
"Yes, I wanted to take a walk this morning."
He reaches for his Russian hat, jokes,
"Do I look like a good comrade?"
"Yes, you do," I say. "Good," from him
and we both laugh, making our way
to the door. I've parked up close,
and I take his arm at the steps.
At times like these I think how
I might have done this with my father
who died at 63; I'm 67 now.
A thin layer of snow covers everything
and we watch our steps, always
fearing a fall. He grabs the car door
and eases himself down. I sigh and

shut the door. We drive through town
past the familiar faces of old buildings.
"Excuse me," he says at the light.
"where is it we're going?"
"To the VA for your blood test, then
on to breakfast at your favorite diner."
"Oh, good," he says, "I should eat something."
"Yes," I say, pulling the car onto the grounds.
"You should and will, right after the test."

We park in the handicapped area
up close to the building, and I get out
thinking through each step. I help
Bill out, steadying him a moment,
then letting him walk on his own.
He refused a cane till he was 90,
didn't want to look like an invalid.
"But what if you fall, Bill?
You'd have to be in a wheelchair."
"Oh," he said, "I'd hate that," and so
he jokes, "I walk on three legs now."

Two old vets greet us at the door,
offer us cookies and coffee. "Thanks,"
I say, shake my head, "Blood test today."
We ride the elevator up to the fourth floor
where the door opens to more old timers

sitting around waiting their turn, brothers and
sisters now, though I have never served.

I go to the check-in desk, while Bill
heads down the hallway, recalling the routine.
I find him sitting by another man
whom I flank in the only open chair.
The hallway is dim and quiet. Men and women
coming and going, many with husbands and wives,
some carrying their clear cup of urine.
Across from us is a chart of military medals.
Bill has several, but doesn't speak of them.
Finally he says to the other man, "Looking round,
I'd say I'm the oldest one here." The man
starts a little, says, "How old are you, sir,
if you don't mind my asking?" I wait.
"Ninety-six," he remembers. I smile then volunteer,
"He was in WW II." The guy turns to Bill,
"What theater?" he asks. "What?" Bill
doesn't hear or understand.
"Where were you stationed?" I translate
loud enough. "Oh, in southern Germany,
part of the occupation army." He could
say more but pauses as a memory awakens.
The guy beside me says, "Sir, I want to thank you
for your service." "What?" Bill asks again.
"He thanks you for your service, Bill." "Oh,"

he sighs, staring at the medal chart, "We had
to stop Hitler." Silence, then a young woman
comes out, calls, "Wright. Wright."
I help him rise again, and we go in.

Leaving the building, Bill lets me
take his arm at the steps. "All this is free,"
he tells me, and I, "You earned it, Bill.
You earned it." Then a few steps from the car,
he stops, takes me by the arm, says, "You know,
helping me like this…you're like the son I lost."
And I swear, I suddenly sense two other men
standing beside us there in morning light, his
Billy grown and aged, and my own lost father.

Moving Bill to the Nursing Home

The letting go of it all,
this sharp pain denied to go on.
The sorting and shifting
of what's left of a life.

Ann and I driving you here,
fixing your photos around the room,
hanging your shirts and pants in a closet,
setting a pillow around your head.
You, Bill, in a nursing home now
drifting toward life's end.
Me acting on your behalf yet
asking where did you go.
My holding the old photos
of you young and younger:
you standing with your father and mother,
with your lovely wife Chris,
you in a WW II uniform,
both of you making a life,
working for what's fair,
marching for what's just.

Old friend, where have you gone to
inside your shrinking body?
I miss our talks, even your

forgetful repetitions.
The sound of your voice
rising like the day to go on.
I sit with you now,
your head bending down,
and I wonder what to say.
Can you hear me still?
Do you understand what's happened?

You are loved, old man.
Look out at the birds
rising outside your window.
See the faces of your neighbors,
all those who touch and lift you
into this day and the next.
You are an old high tree, Bill,
not fallen, but reaching up
and into the sky.

Visiting Bill in the Nursing Home

He lies back all the time now,
has to be roused just to talk.
His eyelids heavy, his heart weak,
his hands just able to hold a cup,
bring trembling bits of food to his lips.
And yet we still can talk
slowly of the day, his life.
"I'm...97," he says as if to explain,
and again I offer, "You're 98, Bill."
as if it's some kind of answer or award.
He's still there inside his body
smiling as best he can, his blue eyes clouded,
his spirit still a low flame.

I used to view my going to his house
as helpful stays with an old friend
who talked his way out of his room
with me seated by his side.
I'd bring him food or take him out
to his favorite diner, Diana's, where
old friends would come and greet him.
I was helping out, hearing history,
learning and laughing along with him.

Now his voice is just above a whisper
hesitating those long seconds
before he's able to think to speak.
I know they care for him well here.
The hospice nurse massages his bare feet,
his thin legs, and cleans his eyes.
Aides tend to his needs now, moving
him about in his padded wheelchair
while I stand back and watch
as they roll him away for lunch.

Before I leave I take his thin hand,
look deep into his blue eyes, "You're 98,"
I say, reminding us both of something.
"I'll be back," I whisper near his face,
Neither of us knowing, each of us
still holding on while letting go.

Taking Bill Home

I.
I ride with Bill by my side,
his physical frailties gone now,
replaced by his ashes. I strap
the box in tight as I would
with him, reach over and
pat him twice, say,
"We're alright, Bill.
I'm driving you home."

As I drive I smile thinking
of how he would enjoy this ride
past the old airport on the bay,
the woods of Sheldon's March where
he loved walking among birds.
I swear "Amazing Grace" is playing
from my car radio—so moving for his passing
that, nearing home, I have to reach over
and turn it off.

At my house, I first carry in
his box of precious photo albums,
then his cartons of clothes
packed caringly by the aides
from the nursing home. Next

I lift him out, about 2 pounds now,
carry him close against my chest.
I call out to my wife, "Honey,
I'm bringing in Bill." Ann comes out
to greet us, her eyes smiling.

We prepare a place for him
above our glassed bookcase.
He is clothed in a velvet bag of
royal purple, a color he never wore,
yet somehow right for him now. We
open bag to find a sealed black box,
a card stating his name and numbers,
simple facts to replace his smile and voice.
Ann asks if we should open the box, and
I stare back through a mute wave of pain.
We do not. We let him rest here
in our home. In a few days we will
journey out together in the weather
to spread him over his beloved lake.

II.
It is Sunday, and we have come
to his old home place where we
will spread our friend's ashes
over an autumn lake. Bright leaves
come floating down to quiet waters.

I kneel along the shore.
Ann says words of blessing as
I cast his dust outwards…
gently falling on soft waves.
Bill's life and mine ripple in the
murky waters before us.
Above—the call of wild geese
winging homeward.

His wife placed here before him,
years ago by his loving hands
now turned to dust in our own.
We stand together in lake wind
holding hands and pouring blessings,
reading his poems of love
as the sun just breaks through
autumn clouds and spreads
its gentle light over all.

Ripening into Age

"The best tunes are played on the oldest fiddles."
–Ralph Waldo Emerson

"No man having drunk old wine desireth new.
For he saith, The old is better."
–Luke 5: 39

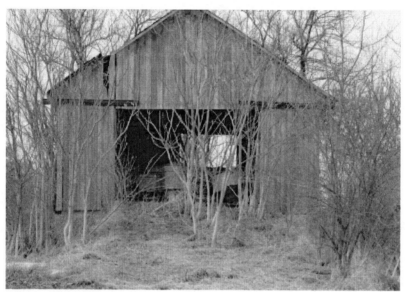
(Photo: Brian Smith)

Growing up in the '50s

We would sit through double features
at the Saturday matinee
my buddies and I breaking
only for trips to the restroom,
nickel candy from the machines,
watching the girls at the popcorn stand.
We'd tolerate the MovieTone newsreel,
less real than our Jungle Jim and the cowboys
fighting and rescuing in the theater dark.
The world we watched we'd carry home
along the streets of our mill town,
shooting out school windows with imagined rifles,
chasing each other over bluffs and ridges.

On mornings, I delivered the papers
reading only the banners:
Pittsburgh Post Gazette, Wheeling Intelligencer,
rolling then dividing them without a mistake.
The news wasn't meant for me.
I craved only the nickel and dime
tips on collection day.
Our first tv taught our parents
to watch the news, and we kids would roll out
to the kitchen to find something to eat,
or sit on the porch watching

for girls in tight shorts.
We'd shoot the breeze as they say
plan fishing trips or walks to the city pool.
Whoever heard of Korea!

By our high school years,
we started doing school reports,
reading up on strange subjects,
copying from encyclopedia,
learning history from photos in books.
It was supposed to make some kind of sense.
"Good, better, best, never let it rest,
Till your good is better, and your better best."
Our civics teacher taught us that,
and I guess we believed it then.

My senior year, reading and watching news
came right after driving and making out.
So I started reading Uncle's *Time* magazine,
believing it our culture's bible, a perhaps
road map away from home.
News, Profiles, Books, Movies, Art—
my circle widened:
Ike would take care of us…
Salk had rescued us from Polio…
The AFL-CIO were now married…

Racial strife met civil rights...
A Communist couple were tried and burned...
The Soviets launched Sputnik, and
Alaska and Hawaii became states.

Knowing things felt like power then,
so I kept up, believing it mattered.
The source of knowledge lay out in space,
replacing any blind faith in God.
College became a Mecca, strange land
where thinking was the ticket.
Friends who opted for jobs
on the railroad, in the steel mills,
selling cars, or enlisting, were
missing out on something grand.
Gradually it happened...
the more I learned,
the less I knew,
and those at the top
knew even less and lived
in denial and lies.
Commerce ran the world.
Philosophy turned in circles.
Science was mere speculation.
Cause and effect separated,
leaving a taste of nausea on the tongue.
Only the world of art mattered.

Reading novels and poems shed
scant light in this darkness.

And then in heat of summer and home,
I fell in love with her and began
learning all over again. Letting go
the reigns of thought alone,
inviting the colors of emotion,
embracing her and life again,
I held them close in the night.
I became that salmon swimming back
upstream and with an open heart.

Back Home in the Valley

Months since I've been back home
to that small town along the river.
Both my parents gone now,
my wife's mother in a nursing home.

I miss the burnt smell of the mill,
the ocean roar of its machines,
the taste of it in the water,
smoke clouds blocking the sky.
Even the old climb the steep hills
from the stores to their homes.
Starlings hang out on telephone lines,
cats run wild between houses.
The street is a parking garage.

And I miss it all, I tell you.
I would walk those streets alone
taking pictures of old houses,
stopping to talk with neighbors,
in the fading light of dusk.

(2009)

Gathering Up

The years pile up then disappear
into the past...like those clothes
hanging at the back of the closet,
passed on to Goodwill. They
come back in old photographs
of what had been...our wedding party
standing on the church steps,
your face a trusting light,
me with a beard, me with hair,
our first dog standing at attention
on the porch where we once lived,
our children small, then growing, then
grown with children of their own.

The years pile up then disappear
inside us, swallowed eggs,
Russian dolls embedded to be
opened with the touch of memory:
the cars we once drove to places
long ago, the rooms and houses
we made our homes, our parents' faces,
their bodies standing near each other,
the special light that falls on all,
a new moon, a new sun.
Who we are. How we go on.

The Water and the Wave

I wake inside the day,
breaking my shell of sleep
into conscious light—
Like a wave my mind
rushes forward on itself
conceiving my script as
somehow separate from myself...
ego crying to be
dressed and fed.

I sense this onward rush yet
pause to measure breath.
My eyes close again—till I feel
the wonder of being just the water.
Harbored in the all,
I do not seek to rise
and be apart from oneness,
and yet...

Sunlight falls through curtains,
a bird calls my name,
my face outside the mirror,
this struggle that is life—
being both water and the wave.

Searching for the Root

The answers lie within, they say, advising how
we become our own path to understanding.

Wet leaves lie across the roadway; strong winds
warn us to stay on the road. And yet
we drive on as though our destination
justifies our blind speed, secretly knowing
we will never quite arrive.

"Where do you feel it in your body?"
my counselor asks, looking down at my hands.
"Can you touch it in yourself?" And I do,
bringing my hands together, then holding
them out before me. "My hands," I say,
"always reaching for something beyond."

She smiles, waits, then nods, "Hostility,"
she tells me, "comes from remembered pain."
And I am struck like a gong by this truth.
Resentment lies underneath my drive
to show and tell them that I'm alright,
and under that I'm holding on
to hurt and unworthiness.

"Breathe in," she whispers, "thinking 'Soo…'"
"Breathe out, with 'Hmm.' Go on try it now."
And I do and I do again, till I feel a lucid
heart release: "Hail, Mary, full of grace."
"May you be filled with loving kindness."
"Peace be with you." All the words
filled now with forgiveness, a touching
and tasting of the wholeness of light.

The answers lie within.

Blessing the Skin

"All creation shares a common skin."
       -Joan Halifax

A friend once told me of how
he could not bear to visit his father
during his last days of cancer,
and I could not understand,
having lost my own good father
sudden and 200 miles away.

And now I've turned away from the
place of my birth, my mother ground,
which seems so wounded:
steel mill town abandoned
of industry—its buildings,
machines and railroad tracks
gone to rust or sold for scrap.
Downtown's become a series
of injuries and scars:
blackened storefronts,
buildings empty or coming down.
The roar of the mill now
a lost echo of better times.
All that I hold in memory and heart
feels used up and gone.

Old men and women walk its streets,
rust scrapes against the skin.

Old town, I want to touch your face,
look close in those eyes and see
what life remains. I bow down
to you and kiss your worn and
weathered skin, listen to your
heart beat, breathe in the
pain and beauty of our age,
ask a blessing on us all.

Alone Looking out the Diner Window

What of those huge empty spaces
inside old factories and steel mills,
high above cold cement floors,
up vacant stairwells near dark roofs
where silence now borders everything?

And what of those huge empty spaces
inside the halls of neighborhood churches,
abandoned pews and school desks
turned over, rain leaking down
and warping old wooden floors?

What of those huge empty spaces
in homes foreclosed, leaving families
to live in cars, bathe in service stations,
kids going to school in dirt-worn clothes
while trying to fit in with the others?

What of those huge empty spaces
inside the hearts of those who have
lost these houses, and jobs, these
marriages and loves and hopes?

And what of these huge empty spaces
in the dream of an America for all?

And how are they to be filled—
by the courage of our children
swallowing hurt, bracing beams,
and opening windows alone?

Charting the Waters

Not from the lakes or streams
but from inside our bodies
said to be 72% water,
the hidden fluid of the self.
It can't be seen from outside,
can't really be tasted or felt,
our essence undisclosed.
All mirrors are false.

In age we may lose some juice,
bend more with wind and weather,
yet our tenderness ripens;
our hands softened to the touch
reach more to embrace.
Forgiveness grows like flowers
blossoming in rain and sun.

The Day Turns

Are you alright?
I ask my friend in her kitchen
and she begins to cry, turns
to tell me, "No one has asked me
that in months."

I enter my son's room
after his divorce and ask,
Are you alright? and he
looks back, holds me with his eyes,
begins to share his anger and his pain.

There are so many ways to be,
so many choices we can make.

My daughter enters the emergency room,
my wife taken upstairs for observation,
and she walks over, touching my arm,
to ask, *Are you alright, Dad?* and I can admit
that I am not.

When my youngest daughter gives birth
to a stillborn child, and my wife
asks weeks later *How are you doing?*
I sit and listen through our tears and doubts,

touch her face to say *I love you.*

> *May you be well.*
> *May you be filled with loving kindness.*
> *May you know your true self.*
> *May you be at peace.*

This is the way we heal and release
the pain of our days.
Leaning into it, we ask
ourselves, then others,
Are you alright?

Are you alright?

Clearing out My Office

No, I've not been fired or let go.
I'm releasing myself after 42 years
of teaching at this college.
Letting go of a career as it were,
using past tense now for the first time.

And I stand alone in this small room
deciding what to save, what to give away,
what to throw in the trash.
Book after book, folder after folder,
knowing I will never teach this again,
yet feeling its weight in memory, in value
given and received from the reading
and conceiving, the sharing together,
the way it can happen in the classroom.
Thousands of faces come streaming back:
some of them eager, some questioning,
some resisting or hardly awake,
all to be opened to the possible.

I've made stacks for the books:
some for the Free Books out in the hall,
some for the library, some special for colleagues,
some for Goodwill, and some so riddled with notes
I think to drop them in the trash, but can't.

They stick in my hands like projects in wood
I've made or carved over the years.
I have always loved books…seen as roadways,
or life savers and ropes to pull one to safety
or out beyond yourself.

I pile the cups and pens and photos
into a box and set it out in the hall,
turn off the computer screen and the light.
I take a breath and close my eyes,
then lug boxes out to the car.

This letting go, a necessary hurt,
is a pain to pass through like birth.
Walking to the car, I smile, knowing that
for all of these years I've been paid
for doing what I love.

Up in the Middle of the Night

Not anxious, just awake, alive
to the pulses within. Thinking
to write something down. Say
something into the void,
the presence in the absence,
the night's quiet.

I hear my dog rustle,
my wife sigh in her sleep,
and I am glad to be
sitting alone, sensing the
sounds of the furnace, the wind,
sound of my own breath.
And then far off and sudden
the call of a train passing in the night
moving towards day.

Into my seventies, I check
my heart rate, the rushing
of blood through my veins.
Thoughts run then walk
slowly towards the dawn.

Too soon all may close forever,
as it did for my father, my mother,

good friends alive now only
in memories. The family Bible
lies under the table, too large
to pick up and read, and yet
inside I know are the stories
of suffering and darkness,
the tests and wisdom gained,
the shining light of love and faith
through darkness and rain.

Tonight I simply listen
to my still beating heart.

Death Echoes

Oh, Bob, my lost brother,
all day I have been searching
for a photo of you.
"Brothers in arms," you once said,
born 4 days apart, you in Brooklyn
I in the Ohio Valley. Each of us
wrote our lives in poems and
stories, yet what united us
was our loving trust in others.

You could sing and play blues guitar,
humbling my own strumming.
While running Carpenter Press you
helped me found Bottom Dog,
each of us somehow doing the work
of our fathers but with words.

I watched you deal with the loss
of your first wife Susan, then
find another in darling Kate.
But it's history now.
I survived my own cancer only to
watch your brave struggle, then passing
from this world in 2007.

And so today, I am feeling your
smile and good laugh as I search
my files and the internet
for an image of you to share. I find
only an old black and white, friend.
My exploring brings little to nothing,
only your last book, *Moving Out,*
Finding Home—strange echo of your life
then and now. *Oh, where have you gone*
my blue-eyed friend? It's a hard rain's
gonna fall. I am seventy now and
need to sit with you on the back porch
sharing our lives as the sun wanes.

In your last days I abandoned you,
your death so near my own.
I should have sat by your side
breathing with you, sharing silence.
I missed this too with my father…death
taking us wherever we are….you and he
hours away, and me hearing on the phone.
Forgive me, my friend, as I forgive myself.

That I can't find signs of you
pains me deeply, for in you I see
my fate. Both of us among the
'notable authors,' neither the great,

nor the remembered. Our real legacy
in the memory of friends and family,
in the faces of our grandkids.

I sat at your service, Bob, watched others
wipe away tears as you sang from your
recordings. I've listened to you sing
again and again, swallowing hard
the pain to be near you. And it doesn't stop
this longing to be with you again as friend.
I call up Kate to ask if she has a photo
she can send me. She promises a couple,
then sighs to tell me, "I can't believe it's been
six years to the day that Bob passed."

Sorrow and release wave over me now
as tears come echoing from my heart.

To a Friend

for Tom

Ann answers the phone from Jen
and gets the news of your death
then repeats it to my numb ears.
My own heart grows tight
and I cannot breathe.

I hold her in tears a long while, then
move out to the garage where I
pull the lawnmower out
from the rubble of bikes and tarps.
I will pace my emotion with work.

I begin going up and down the yard
eating the grass with a noisy machine.
I want to lie down in a grass of tears
but go on, working it.

I overhear my neighbor
talking with the Chem-Lawn people
going to kill off her bugs and weeds.
I know that you refused the Emergency Room
because you lacked health insurance, and so
I grow angry at all those who value
lawn care over the healthcare.

I turn my anger at loss to others,
as I do with the news of war,
job losses, gas prices.

I have to push through the high grass
out back, and I feel incredibly tired
sweating the pain of it all, taking each step
as it comes.

It is two days later and I have been
facing your loss a moment at a time,
opening the door to it, remembering
your wildness, your kindness,
your imagination, your laughter.

At your funeral we greet others,
offer up stories or your life,
and, though I see your dead face a few feet away,
I sense you are with us still
in our love and pain. I mean really, Tom,
what would we do without you?

Awakening

She turns in bed and
releases a soft moan,
finding comfort in her dreams.
I lie there thinking of her skin,
the warmth of her thighs, soft lips
pressed firm into mine.
A moment away from touch,
I listen again for her breath.
To waken this flower
is to dance in water,
to sing with our bodies
of love that survives.

These Days

We rise early just before dawn
and spread our blanket on the floor
for gentle yoga practice. Ann smiles
quietly as we lie back, our bodies
spread out like plants on the earth.
I start the practice video, move into position
and begin to breathe deep and slow,
lifting my arms above my head
then down to my sides, over and over
yet slowly. "Be the tortoise," she says.
Our dog comes over to inspect,
sniffs at my face, lays her head down
on my chest. "Not now," I say yet rest
thankful to be blessed by this gentle
work, this body alive and stretching,
this sun rising, this woman I love.

Night Call

This evening on Lummi Island
we sit among tall trees, along
the shores of Bellingham Bay.
Ann and I, the older couple
at breakfast, here among the
twilight songs of birds.

Our daughter's family is safe
in their cabin nearby,
and so we two from Ohio
sit in a native hot tub
gazing out through hushed firs
as the sun so beautifully sets.

I touch her smooth leg
beneath the water
and she smiles into a kiss.
The water surrounds us, as we
breathe the sweet scent
of this moment, all of it
gently touched by the knowing
that this dear life of ours
does not go on forever.

When I Am 70...It's Time

Well, this large number sounds so
rounded and aged, but not like wine.
"Well, he's in his 70s," they'll say
as if surprised I can still tie my shoes.
I used to tell people to get things done
before they're in their 80s. Now
I'm at that stage. "Hurry up, it's time,"
the barman says about to close,
but I want to stand long and
enjoy the last drinks. Not take off
into the dark night of oblivion
or heaven, whichever comes next....
If our gone parents could but talk.
I so love my wife, sons and daughters,
the whole family of grandkids. I love
watching them grow and change,
finding themselves again and again,
friends whose faces echo lives.
I love making music, putting words to
head and heart, sharing them, or
sitting still not measuring anything,
watching the candle slowly burn,
talking close with Ann, remembering,
tasting the food of life. Oh,
how can I ever give this up?

Working Out

Sweating on the treadmill and
staring out the large window
at snow falling on the parking lot
where cars glide around on ice,
I breathe hard this work of
bringing my body whole again.
In seven days I will be seventy-one,
a large number for anyone to count.
Last week my granddaughter who's five
jumped from sixty-eight, sixty-nine,
back to twenty-one. Bless her.

Is that what I am doing, sweating off
the years I've built up, like taking time
to clean out the garage or basement?
I grip the handle bar, take a breath,
and step into it, again and again,
wanting to be there as these children
gently age.

The Taste

"No man also having drunk old wine desireth new:
for he saith, The old is better." Luke 5: 39

And I have become the old wine,
aged, full, yet clearer. And though
the taste of age is sometimes bitter,
it is also more true to the vine.

This is not boasting, but listening
to the strains of my life. Enjoying
the sounds of children running
in a schoolyard, the face of a
young mother lifting her child,
eyeing the father waiting
for his daughter to exit the bus.
Workers bending forward
into their job, laughing
with the weight of it.
Sisters and brothers
wiping the brow of another.

One can see and know all this
in quiet or go blindly about the day,
wasting the warmth and light.
I hear the world's sorrow

in the newspaper, yet don't
subscribe to it. There is
so much good to taste.
Today I smile at sunrise and sunset,
lift the glass of life overfull.

Walking a Field into Evening

For learned books, I read the grasses.
For reputation, a bird calls my name.
I cross a stone bridge with the pace of dusk.
At the meadow gate, six cows meditate.

For decades I ran my mind up hill and down;
now idleness tells me what is near.
An arrow of wild geese crosses the sky,
my body still, my feet firm on the ground.

We age like trees now, watch our seedlings
take wind or grow around us.
I'm going to mark my books lightly
with a pencil. When someone wants
to take my picture, I'll walk towards them
and embrace.

No more arguments,
just heart sense, or talk about nothing.
Take long walks in the woods at dawn and dusk,
breathe in the damp musty air,
learn to listen before I die.

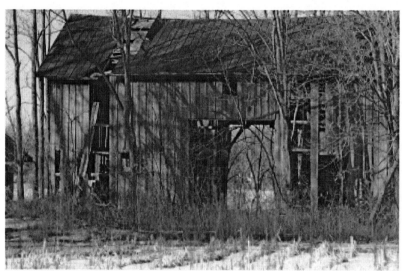

Photo: Brian Smith

Finding Faith

"To fear is to expect punishment. To love is to know we are immersed, not in darkness, but in light."
- Mother Teresa

"All I have seen teaches me to trust the Creator for all I have not seen."
- Ralph Waldo Emerson

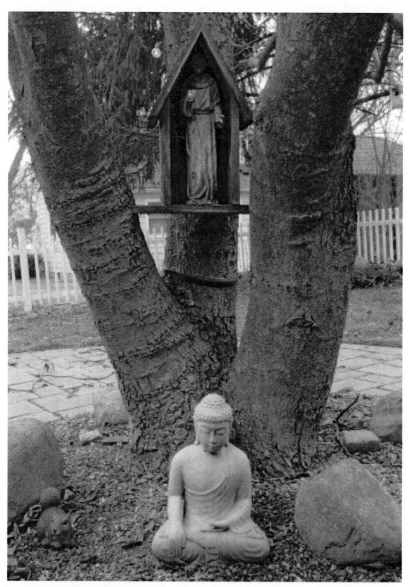

(Smith backyard, photo: Larry Smith)

My Journey Home

I.

Sitting in a front pew of the Potter
Memorial Presbyterian Church,
I wait for my father and uncle
to join me and my brother.
I am 14 years old, a freshman,
and have just come up from
the basement Sunday school.
For long moments I stare up
at the mural painting of Christ
in the Garden of Gethsemane.
In ten minutes the church will almost fill,
and the robed choir will rise slowly to sing,
proclaiming God's love for all.

> "I am weak, but thou art strong.
>
> Jesus, keep me from all wrong.
>
> I'll be satisfied as long
>
> as I walk, dear Lord, close to thee…"

None of this is new to me, yet
something strange is happening here, as I
stare up at Christ kneeling in the garden,
God's light breaking through darkness.
I close my eyes and whisper to myself and God,

> *If you are truly here, God, give me a sign,*
>
> *make Yourself present to me.*

I am bold yet shaken by this challenge.
At last month's revival, I sat and did
not make the altar call.

The hymn has ended and the minister
stands large before me reading the Gospel.
He raises his arms, extends his open palms
pouring out God's love and grace.
I close my eyes and feel it all
washing over me. A stillness comes to
steal my breath. My body quivers,
my brother moves away. My father
looks down on me sitting there
while others now are standing.
"Are you alright, son?" he asks, and I
shake my head, whisper "I'm going to be sick,"
"Go," he says, "Now." And I do, rushing out
past the others praying the Our Father...
    Our Father, my father...

The way home is a blur...past houses and cars,
yards and flowers, up the hill where I
burst through the door, gasping, trembling.
Mother comes towards me from the kitchen,
"What's wrong, honey?" she asks, bending
towards my face. "My God," she sighs,
stroking my hair, "you're whiter than a ghost."

"No, I'm okay," I say and run out and up
the stairs to my room. I throw myself
onto my unmade bed, breathing through tears.
My heart beats strong inside my chest and head.
Love and fear have a hold of me.
I will lie there in God's grace for an hour,
and when I rise, I will tell no one.

II.
Sitting in Brown Chapel at
Muskingum Presbyterian College,
I am humbled by the choir which
rivals even the huge pipe organ
shaking the room into abeyance.
A freshman again, I watch and listen,
afraid of failing my family and class.
Attendance is taken by older peers
as we sit prayerful twice a week.

By midterms, our religious roots
have transplanted to science, math,
literature, and art. Other ways of seeing,
other ways of being. Let them take roll,
we are free to think on our own.
My attention turns to watching co-eds
in the library, smooth legs under
open trench coats. "A small Christian college

for small Christians," someone says,

and one by one we drift outward

onto a lake of doubt or unbelief.

III.

Love enters my life, teaching me;

soon she and I take classes to wed

in St. Agnes Catholic Church,

sessions with a young priest where

we listen, smile, and nod.

Ann's father walks her down the aisle

in tears, my family sitting on the right side,

unable to kneel at an unfamiliar altar.

We will raise our children in the Church

while they attend public schools. We

compromise our beliefs, and so we sit

as family during mass, I watching the faces

of others take the wafer onto their tongues.

A lover of literature, I read my spiritual light

deep in the Transcendentalists: Emerson and

Thoreau my private saints. Whitman and Dickinson

lights unto themselves. Each summer

I pilgrimage to Concord and Walden Pond

to walk Nature's path under trees of light.

IV.

Now 50 at Mt. Tremper Buddhist Temple
in upstate New York, I just sit
staring at the wooden floor boards—
bird sounds in the approaching dark.
Stillness fills the room as we walk
mindful of our steps and breath.
In the dark we learn to feel our way
back to our cabins and bunks. Blinded
by our own light, each day we learn
to sit inside the moment, soft breath
of trees and sky. No God to answer to, no
list of sins and commandments,
intuition beyond reason, luminous
from within the heart space.
Newly awakened I will drive this home.

V.

Almost 70 now and retired, a
sitting Catholic for 45 years, I
swallow my lack of trust to embrace
the beauty of Christian faith. I rise
from my seat to attend classes,
sense the rich texture of the Word,
the depth of contemplation.
I make a witness before others.
To some I am a convert, to myself

I'm who I've always been, the circle
grown outward toward infinity.
We still sit with friends in meditation,
welcome others in where more and
more I sense God's grace everywhere
in everything, everyone. The Church
exists imperfect inside the light of God.

At Easter time I take the host and wine
into myself…feel it soften in my mouth
and throat. I am one with it wholly.
Like a salmon swimming back upstream,
I have made the long journey home.

Calling and Receiving

for Richard Rohr

And how do I speak to you of a faith
confirmed by all that exists? Inner and
outer worlds made one in awareness.
The long embrace of diversity.
Union of life's mysteries.
Finding God inside us, and
ourselves in God. Living and
loving this moment before us.

Oh, long river of awareness—
not pushing or grasping it,
not wanting all to swim
or to call it by the same name,
but drowning in it again
and again, swallowing old self,
going in and under to rise
and find true ground again.

Winter Solstice along the Lake

The sacred scripture of the earth. –Fionntulach

My wife and I rise at 6 a.m.
and walk the dog down dark streets
in cool lake air, past yards and houses,
lit only by distant streetlamps.

Near the lake we stop to
sense the dark's deep mystery,
breathe it in, eyes closed
or open the same.
"Advent time," I feel and say.
"Yes," she whispers back,
"before the birthing of light."
The dog pulls on her leash.

At the shoreline,
our footsteps further the darkness,
as we still, sounds grounding us now,
the quiet roll of the lake's black waters,
our bodies' deep sense of space and time.
And there to the east
above the line of earth
beneath soft hanging clouds
glows a soft purple aura,

maternal curve of light,
the birthing crown.

The dog stills at our feet.
My arms wrap around my wife
as we breathe life's circle,
allow earth's sweet light to come.

Converging Paths

I.
We find an old building
in downtown Sandusky
and rent floor space
for sitting twice a month.

Two couples opening
a dharma center
in the Midwest.

We order black zafu cushions
for sitting, craft a screen
and wooden altar.

We make space for it
in our lives
invite our friends
to share the quiet.

II.
Converging Paths
is our name for it,
a center where we come
to stretch and sit,
breathe silence together.

We've chosen the labyrinth
as symbol, the one from Chartres
that slowly winds into itself
in darkness and light.

And so we come from diverse ways
into one, a union of acceptance,
unforced yet discovered,
as though we've all arrived
at the same anonymous station.

Not destination, but pathways
we've found within ourselves.

Embracing Old Codes

Namaste
I see the light in you…
love thy neighbor as thyself.
I see the light in you.

It all echoes.
It all rings
like a great
gong of peace.

May you be filled
with loving-kindness
May you be well.
May you be peaceful
and at ease.
May you be happy.

The circle extends,
all life taken in.
The circle extends,
all life taken in.

Do unto others
as you would have them
do unto you.

My father's code:
If you can't say something
good about another,
say nothing at all.

Non-judgment
non-duality
the heart space.

I see the light in you.

In the Rectory Office

"How do you see God," she asks me,
the gentle nun in plain clothes
sitting across a table from me.
And I am unable to answer at first,
so she looks direct into my eyes,
"How did you see God as a child?"
I shy away from Hollywood visions
of the old sky God with long beard
and flowing white robe. I stare back
 say, "What comes is the image of Jesus
gathering the children to him,
a mural painting in our Sunday School.
It was larger than life and warmed
that bare Presbyterian classroom."

She sits and nods as I say,
"A larger one at the church front
was of Jesus-God at Gethsemane
kneeling alone at the dark rocks,
a warm light above blessing him."
She smiles at this, and I do not tell her
how I stared at it while the minister spoke on,
or how I watched the pretty girl with
dark hair and eyes in the choir.
"God was Jesus, and Jesus, God.
The two were one to me then," I confess.

"Isn't that why He was sent?"
She nods her head gently, says, "Yes,
and tell me how do you see God now?"

Again I grow quiet, confusion reigns
in my heart, a stream I must cross to speak.
Questions of suffering block me, and
no sharp image appears. And then…
it falls from my lips, "God is everywhere,
in everything, in everyone. God is just
this space, this presence we awaken to."
Her eyes too open at this saying
that unites us and all.
A quiet falls over us…a long stillness
that we drink together there.

And finally I hear myself say,
"You know, each morning as I
pull out of my neighborhood, I
look across the road into a wide schoolyard,
and it's just full of children running and
playing together in the sun."
She touches my hand and smiles.
I breathe deep.

Just Practice

"And who told you that meditating
was not a form of prayer?"
Buddha asks us.

"And who is it told you
that you were naked?"
God asks of Adam.

The things we tell ourselves
without question are blocks
on our pathway. All thought
is not truth.

And when we sit or pray
in simple practice, we do so
without judgment, in acceptance.
If we watch closely for a sign,
again we block our way.
Just sit. Breathe in and out,
with it here and now
and for all time.

Let Be

You deal with it.
Don't bury it with answers.
Work with it, a breath
at a time. Hold it
in your diaphragm—
not in and out—
hold it right there,
burning hot in your gut.
Your problems won't change;
only you will.
Break open the egg of you
and cook with compassion.
Don't rush. Let go,
and let be.

Those who judge quickly
sacrifice seeing for belief.
"Accept the shadow," they say
"for the real." I too and perhaps you
sink into this vision under water,
our eyes clouded with sedge,
our ears muted with clay
to all that lives and breathes
in the bright light of day.

Sitting with Him at the Meditation Center

We sit together on cushions,
the sun setting outside the windows,
our room full of soft candle light.

> *May I be filled with loving kindness.*
> *May I be well.*
> *May I be peaceful and at ease.*
> *May I be happy.*

This wish for ourselves and world
leans us forward into our days.

Our silence wraps around us
as we begin this night
bringing the faces of others
we have feared and loved before us,
sending Metta love to all.

> *May you be filled with loving kindness*
> *May you be well.*
> *May you be peaceful and at ease.*
> *May you be happy.*

Gently guided I bring forth
the face of my father

gone now twenty-five years:
rugged brows in the rounded face
of a worker, his dark earnest eyes
neither asking nor answering—
my heart, my heart, my throat, my eyes,
soft tears within my breath.

> *With each breath the heart opens.*
> *With each breath the mind returns.*

I have passed him now with my years
and see his strong-soft face
as the friend he has become.

> *May we be filled with loving kindness.*

Mary's Feet

Outside the retreat center
I walk the green grounds
pausing at a meditation bench,
the stone grotto, a fallen oak
among the pines.

Slowly I circle the nun's cemetery
following the Stations of the Cross,
small brick pillars holding the
metal plaques of the crucifixion.
And I am moved as always
by Christ's sacrifice, the slow
steady movement toward death
then resurrection—pain and
love shared in each.

I pass more towering pine
stepping softly over tender grass,
then sit upon a cedar bench.

There across from me is a stone statue
of Mary among the flowers—
her face beautifully kind as always.
She calms my breath with quietness,
and for the first time I see—

her bare feet beneath the robe,

her toes bent and human

as my own.

Morning Practice

My guitar leans on the glider
waiting to be stroked and sung to.
Too early for sleeping neighbors,
I sit and feel the coming light.
My dog barks to be let out,
then dashes across wet grass.
Sunlight plays across the back fence
as the chatter of birds comes clear.
The cardinal's awakening song:
Whoit-Whoit-Purdy-Purdy-Purdy
tells me life is here, in each breath,
each breeze, each smell of spring green.
This time as dawn comes on,
we receive what we accept
within the light.

Naming the Mind

And so we sit together,
yet enter the stillness privately,
listening with each breath,
not denying the world, but
opening to its mystery.
We are naming the mind,
the breath rising and falling,
this slow allowing,
words dropping into the stream
and fading into light.
This new freedom we share,
great gift we haven't to earn,
this quiet grace of caring
spread with the breath over
all that is or ever was.

None stand outside this
prayer that we all are.

Receiving

"My deepest me is God."
- St. Catherine of Genoa

I think of no answers, no questions,
just this serene acceptance of rivers,
flowing deep presence.

Step into the movement
without a voice or a name.

Go further, deeper, trusting
the grace of poverty and nakedness.

We stumble to rise, find ourselves afloat
in the gaze of God's love.

With One Voice

Waking the birds inside my guitar,
I pick and strum, glide fingers over strings,
touch their feathers tenderly.
Oh, let the birds begin.

Beginning to play years ago
I strained sore fingers for chords,
beat a savage rhythm, hearing
without listening, volume high,
the way I would toot my cornet,
hitting notes not songs.

After years of playing and soft listening,
I've learned to love what comes,
not make sounds of darkness,
but bend to it, blend body with it,
dance it along, touch and release—
Oh, listen to the birds sing.

Dreaming of Guitars and Voices

Last night I was dreaming in notes of music,
black dots in a field of light
that I could see and hear in my sleep.
The songs were the new hymns I'd
learned from playing in church:
"pa-ra...con-stru-ir...la...co-mun-i-dad!"
"O Love of God" strummed with force,
picked with conviction. I watched
black notes appear as the melody
rang out. Someone else was
helping me play the notes...
the way God's spirit at Mass
moves my fingers lightly over strings,
lifting me and others in true song
from page into air—
"O Love of God, gather us...

      that we may share...

           the gifts we are given."
"pa-ra...con-stru-ir...la...co-mun-i-dad!"

Sitting with the Choir

The lights are dim as others
drift in, finding their places.
Families slide into pews
with hardly a sound.
Soft Easter candles speak all.

The choir rises to sing.
I strum the guitar as the organ
spreads music like a gentle rain
over everything.

A priest walks among us
casting water from a sprig of pine
onto bowed or upturned faces,
his footsteps followed by a
white robed altar boy and girl.

And then one hand passes to another
a small candle flame, till light spreads
to full illumination. Again the choir
rises to call forth song as I gently strum:
"Rock of Ages…cleft for me.
Let me hide…myself in Thee."
Old Protestant hymns moving the mass.

The Mass Has Begun

I play the guitar, look over at the choir
singing strong and clear, their voices
ringing like church bells calling us.
A white flow of altar boys and girls
prepares the way for our priest in
his robe of white and green.
Joined to this welcome I bow
to the notes before me, listen close
to the Sister's piano playing
setting rhythm and pace:
"We are one in the Spirit.
We are one in the Lord."

Standing in the Light

Sitting in church and
strumming the final chord
of the hymn, I look up
for approval…at whom?
God…the congregation…my father?
And why do I desire it, need it so,
always hope it will come? I've
been slave to approval most
of my life—a mother who
praised me too easily, a
father who didn't know how.
His father gave him none.

Leaning on a shovel, having
put all the tools away, I'd look
around and he'd be gone
onto another task. His to give
but he didn't know. No blame
or shame is attached here.
May I shed some praise on
my own family. In my 70s
enter this forgiving light.

The Transformation

For the last two Sundays at Mass
I have looked deep into the host
as the priest holds it high
before the congregation.
I have looked with all myself to
feel the transubstantiation.
His words and the sounds of others
all melt away before the thought,
Is this the body and blood of Christ?
For this moment all life rests on this.
For years I have accepted it
as symbol and rite. "Do this in
remembrance of me." And I have thought,
What greater way to enter Christ than by
taking Him into your body. And yet today
in this moment as he holds it high in light,
something quietly moves in me, connecting me
to the host in a way I've never felt. A glow
radiates from it. *Is the host now Christ*
or is it I who am transformed,
brought into a new way of seeing
and being with God? A hush falls over me
as I kneel, then lift my head in song,
"Amazing Grace, how sweet thou art....
I once was blind, but now I see."

This Cold Sunday Morning

Having risen with the birds, I am
using the church envelope as a marker
in a book of poems about faith and doubt.
Frost again on the car's window shield,
snow piled high on everything.

What makes me rise to wash and
dress for church lies deep inside.
Perhaps the quiet light of candles,
the company of others gathered
near the altar: their faces, bodies
sitting and rising, slowly moving forward.
All of this unspoken, as we prepare the meal
of body and blood with the words, our song
lifted up, our deep intention to be present.

Yes, children rustle in their pews, a baby
cries and is taken out, an altar boy
gets confused, but it is all a dance
of gentle acceptance, ours and His.
A communion wafer melts in wine
at the back of the throat, as I sigh
and swallow life.

Walking in Water

I have been trying to talk with God—
honestly seeking a voice to speak with Him.
I've managed it with Mary and Jesus,
though the specter of His dying and rising
leaves me speechless. But God
is just so beyond yet of it all,
the beginning and end of being.
Now I see that what I am
really doing is trying to pray.
I want to believe that I can.
I want to do more than nod or bow.
I am dying to be with Him.

Today in the motel swimming pool
I stood and closed my eyes, just
sensing the slow pulsing of water
against my skin, the liquid mystery
of it so godlike, and I am in and of it:
the way of water—liquid baptism
—and so of the air, soft breath we all share.

I begin to speak soft words to God
asking His help in forgiving others,
asking His forgiveness for myself.

"Lord, I've been so slow in coming,
not answering the door, making
my own house to rival Yours.
In Your grace, grant us mercy."
I open my eyes, feel water and air
surround me, His great
heart of being.

Wearing Grace

> "Christ has no body now on earth but yours."
> -Theresa of Avila

I wear a mala bracelet now
of wooden beads wrapped close
around my naked wrist. Echo
of all religions' humbleness.
Reminder of the paths within
which hold and whisper grace.
A simple presence, all and nothing,
wooden beads carved by machines,
stained an earthy brown, and strung by
hands somewhere in Singapore or
Bangladesh. I touch each bead, hold
or roll its hardness with simple intention,
each a bone, a rounded stone.
I whisper prayers of loving-kindness
or hail Mary, full of grace, all of it
ever present and lower case.

When We Walk

Walking slow and gently
around the meditation room,
or through the cool yard grass,
or down the sidewalk of our neighborhood
or along a row of city buildings
we walk for many.
For those who cannot walk:
lying in their hospital beds,
or sitting up in wheelchairs,
for those so loaded down with struggle
they feel they cannot freely walk.
We take each step, each measured breath,
kiss the ground with foot bottoms.
A child again, we walk the earth.

The Old Farmer's Way

He works his garden now
with his back and hoe,
bending and lifting, watering
most mornings as the sun
falls on tender leaves.

When his minister asked him,
"Silas, do you pray as you work?"
he paused to stroke his graying beard.
"I guess I see my work as prayer,"
he spoke into the minister's face.
The farmer, not a man of words,
spread his hands to the green,
then reading the puzzled look—
"I sow and they do the growing."
The minister smiled, "But do you not
offer prayer for good weather?"
The farmer shook his head and
looked off to the end of the field,
"You got to accept what comes."
The minister paused, "And are you
not thankful of your yield?"
Once more he shook his head, said low, "Ah,
that's where the prayer comes in."

Who Speaks for God?

Who says that it was
all meant to happen?
The pain caused to children,
the cutting people off,
an anguish for others or
losing all in a storm
of fire or rage?

Who speaks for this
as God's divine plan
lays on others a cross
they have not made
or earned or sought.

Only courage through pain,
love through our losses,
and a hope beyond our sorrows
allows us to endure.

What Is Given

"…knowing no effort earns
that all-surrounding grace."

-Denise Levertov

The difference between belief and faith is a
knowing trust. One is thought and measured,
the other felt and endless. *Oh, net of being
hidden in plain sight: the air, the light, the river's flow,
ever changing growth of day and night.* We touch
and know a story greater than we can understand.
We taste its bitter sweetness, feel its cool burning in our throat;
we close our eyes to see: one breath—one body.
Taught to hold back the individual, we fought faith,
yet now surrender to an all beyond self that is
yet one with it. We wear the clothes of others,
taste forgiveness on our breath.
Open eyes, open heart, to what is given.

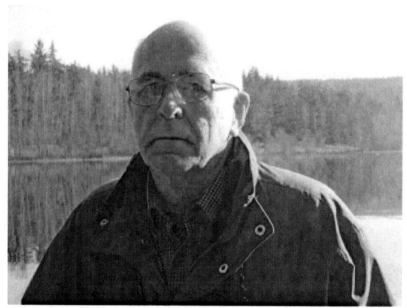

(Larry Smith 2014, photo: Laura Smith)

Larry Smith is a native Midwesterner, born and raised in a working-class family in the industrial Ohio River Valley. In 1965 he graduated from Muskingum Colleg in Ohio and at 21 married a hometown girl, Ann Zaben. He worked in the steel mills that summer and they soon moved to Euclid, Ohio where he taught high school and Ann began working as a nurse. He earned degrees at Kent State University (M.A. and Ph.D), and was there when the riots and shootings of students occurred. In 1970-1971 he and Ann and their daughter Laura moved to Huron, Ohio where he began teaching at Firelands College of Bowling Green State University and had two children, Brian and Suzanne. In 1980 he and family traveled to Sicily where he was a Fulbright lecturer in American Literature.

He is the author of eight books of poetry, a book of memoirs, five books of fiction, two literary biographies of authors Lawrence Ferlinghetti and Kenneth Patchen, and two books of translations from the Chinese with co-translator Mei Hui Huang. His photo history of his hometown *Mingo Junction* appeared recently in the Images of America Series. Two of his film scripts on authors James Wright and Kenneth Patchen have been made into films with Tom Koba and shown on PBS. As a professor of English and humanities at Firelands College (1970-2012) he has taught writing and literature and served as director of the Firelands Writing Center, a cooperative of writers. As director of the literary publisher, Bottom Dog Press, Inc., he has edited over 60 books and carried into publication some 170 titles of poetry, fiction, and nonfiction. He and Ann with Jan and Lou Young founded the Converging Paths Meditation Center in Sandusky, Oh.

Smith is a consultant for Wayne State University Press, and has been a reviewer for *American Book Review, Parabola, Small Press Review, Choice, The San Francisco Review of Books, The Columbus Dispatch, Ohioana Quarterly, Heartlands,* and the *New York Journal of Books.* He is a requested presenter at various writers' conferences in Ohio, Michigan, Pennsylvania, and Kentucky. His poetry has been featured on American Public Media's *Writer's Almanac* with Garrison Keillor. His novel *The Free Farm* was released in 2012 from Bottom Dog Press. He and his wife Ann live along the shores of Lake Erie in Huron, Ohio.

BOTTOM DOG PRESS
BOOKS IN THE HARMONY SERIES

Lake Winds: Poems
By Larry Smith 218 pgs. $18
An Act of Courage: Selected Poems of Mort Krahling
Eds. Judy Platz & Brooke Horvath, 104 pgs. $16
On the Flyleaf: Poems
By Herbert Woodward Martin, 104 pgs. $16
The Stolen Child: A Novel
By Suzanne Kelly, 350 pgs. $18
The Canary: A Novel
By Michael Loyd Gray, 192 pgs. $18
The Harmonist at Nightfall: Poems of Indiana
By Shari Wagner, 114 pgs. $16
Painting Bridges: A Novel
By Patricia Averbach, 234 pgs. $18
Ariadne & Other Poems
By Ingrid Swanberg, 120 pgs. $16
The Search for the Reason Why: New and Selected Poems
By Tom Kryss, 192 pgs. $16
Kenneth Patchen: Rebel Poet in America
By Larry Smith, Revised 2nd Edition, 326 pgs. Cloth $28
Selected Correspondence of Kenneth Patchen,
Edited with introduction by Allen Frost,
312 pgs. Paper $18/ Cloth $28
Awash with Roses: Collected Love Poems of Kenneth Patchen
Eds. Laura Smith and Larry Smith
With introduction by Larry Smith, 200 pgs. $16
* * * *

HARMONY COLLECTIONS AND ANTHOLOGIES
Come Together: Imagine Peace
Eds. Ann Smith, Larry Smith, Philip Metres, 204 pgs. $16
Evensong: Contemporary American Poets on Spirituality
Eds. Gerry LaFemina and Chad Prevost, 240 pgs. $16
America Zen: A Gathering of Poets
Eds. Ray McNiece and Larry Smith, 224 pgs. $16
Family Matters: Poems of Our Families
Eds. Ann Smith and Larry Smith, 232 pgs. $16

Bottom Dog Press, Inc.
PO Box 425/ Huron, Ohio 44839
http://smithdocs.net

CPSIA information can be obtained at www.ICGtesting.com
Printed in the USA
LVOW05s1101020514

384204LV00001B/50/P